RESTARTING
WORKBOOK AND FACILITATOR´S GUIDE

FOR USE WITH THE RESTARTING DVD SERIES
TWELVE WEEKS COURSE WORKBOOK
Ed Khouri

PART OF
THRIVING: *RECOVER YOUR LIFE*

Shepherd's House Inc.
P.O. Box 40096
Pasadena, CA 91114

www.lifemodel.org
www.thrivingrecovery.org

© 2007 by Edward M. Khouri Jr.

Published by Shepherd's House Inc.
P.O. Box 40096
Pasadena, CA 91114
www.lifemodel.org

All rights reserved. No part of this publication may be reproduced, stored in a retrieval system, or transmitted in any form or by any means – for example, electronic, photocopy, recording – without the prior written permission of the publisher. The only exception is brief quotations in printed reviews.

ISBN number 978-0-9674357-3-2

KJV Scripture quotations are from: The Holy Bible: King James Version. 1995. Logos Research Systems, Inc.: Oak Harbor, WA.

NKJV Scripture quotations are from: The New King James Version. 1996, 1982, Thomas Nelson: Nashville.

NIV Scripture quotations are from: The Holy Bible, NEW INTERNATIONAL VERSION®. Copyright 1973, 1978, 1984 International Bible Society. All rights reserved throughout the world. Used by permission of International Bible Society.

RSV Scripture quotations are from: The Revised Standard Version. 1971, Logos Research Systems, Inc.: Oak Harbor, WA.

Good News Bible Scripture quotations are from: *The Good News Bible*. 1966, 1971, 1976, American Bible Society: New York, NY.

The Message Scripture quotations are taken from: *The Message*. Copyright 1993, 1994, 1995, 1996, 2000, 2001, 2002. Used by permission of NavPress Publishing Group.

The Twelve Steps are quoted from: *The Anonymous Press Mini-Edition* of Alcoholics Anonymous. The Anonymous Press, 1992, 2005. The inclusion of the Twelve Steps does not mean that A.A. has reviewed or approved the contents of this publication, nor that A.A. agrees with the views expressed in the Restarting video. A.A. is a program of recovery from alcoholism only. Use of the Twelve Steps in contents and discussions which address other matters does not imply otherwise.

Dr. Daniel Amen:
Change Your Brain, Change Your Life, New York, NY: Random House, 1998.
Healing The Hardware Of The Soul, New York, NY: Simon & Schuster, Inc., 2002.

Dr. Allan Schore:
Affect Regulation and the Origin of the Self, Hillsdale, NJ: Erlbaum, 1994.
Affect Regulation And The Repair Of The Self, New York, NY: W. W. Norton & Company, 2003.
Dysregulation And Disorders Of The Self, New York, NY: W. W. Norton & Company, 2003.

TABLE OF CONTENTS

Thanks and Acknowledgements 4

Forward 5

Welcome to Restarting 7
    A Revolution of Hope
    How Can I Use My Workbook?
    God and Restarting

Restarting Group Ground-rules 12

CHAPTER 1 Train Your Brain for Change! 15

CHAPTER 2 The 2 Skills Your Brain Can't Live Without 23

CHAPTER 3 Calming Our Painful Emotions 33

CHAPTER 4 Strategies That Keep You Stuck 41

CHAPTER 5 Healthy Relationships 53

CHAPTER 6 Painful Relationships 67

CHAPTER 7 Toxic Relationships 83

CHAPTER 8 Trauma, Hope and Recovery 95

CHAPTER 9 Leaving Codependency Behind 107

CHAPTER 10 Attachments That Kill: How Addictions Re-wire Your Brain ... 119

CHAPTER 11 Recovering Our Lost Identity 133

CHAPTER 12 The Blueprint for a New You! 145

Facilitator Notes 161
    What is Restarting?
    How is each Restarting lesson organized?
    What is included in the weekly Restarting DVD lessons?
    What do I need to facilitate a Restarting group?
    What kind of meeting place do I need?
    What are the ground-rules that can help keep my group safe?
    What else do I need to know that will help me facilitate Restarting?

Facilitator Chapter Overviews 173

ACKNOWLEDGEMENTS

This workbook – and the Restarting project – would not be possible without the help, encouragement and joyful support from many people.

Maritza, you are my joy, love and partner in life. Aside from the fact that you have the most beautiful curly hair and smile of anyone I know, you gave up time with me, and sacrificed what you wanted so that this workbook could be complete. Your input, advice, ideas, creativity and expertise are woven throughout this workbook in patterns that most people will never know. We share the hope that many will be able to walk fully into the joy, life and recovery that we experience together. Your support, care and understanding are what made it possible for me to finish. Thank you, Bellisima!

Jim, you are a blessing. This workbook and project could have never happened without you. The Life Model has changed how I view life and recovery, and it has enriched the relationship that Maritza and I share. Your wisdom, discernment, editing, patience, kindness and boundless joy have fueled this project. When we started out, I never dreamed what Thriving and Restarting could become. It is fun to dream with you!

Jake and Jordan, thanks for giving me the time to write. You are joys to me, and it is my hope that you will walk fully into the destiny that God has placed within your heart.

Deni, you have helped me mature and grow in ways I never knew possible. You are such a delight! You make me proud to be your dad every day.

Chris, you bring me hope for the next generation of recovery leaders.

Tucker, you are truly the Thriving Dog!

Thanks to the Equipping Hearts Board and Vision Team for your support, encouragement and practical advice.

Karl and Charlotte, thank you so much for your gentleness, compassion, faithfulness and perseverance. You never gave up - and never stopped seeking the presence of Jesus. He has given you something extraordinary to share with the world, and thanks to your hard work, the lives of many hurting people are going to be transformed forever through Immanuel Process moments.

Mom and Dad, thanks for loving me enough to teach me to do my best – and to do hard things. You taught me a standard of excellence that has remained with me throughout my life.

I have been blessed with the friendship of many who have taught and mentored me over the years, and to you I am deeply grateful. Thanks to Brian McLaren, Don and Patty Isaac, Jim Isom, Dee Bissel, Mickey Evans and the folks at Dunklin Memorial Camp, Dave Erickson, Ron Ross, Charles and Jean LaCour, David Partington, Alan Smith, Steve Watson, Chris and Jen Coursey, and Bob Jones. There is a part of you all in this project.

FOREWORD

I am a person in recovery from the pain of trauma and addictions. I know from personal experience what it feels like to be stuck in the pain and shame of life-controlling problems – and not be able to break free. I think this paraphrase from the book of Lamentations describes it best:

How deserted I feel.
I once had friends and people around me, but now I am alone.
My life once mattered to me and to others – my dreams were important,
But now I have become a slave.

I cry – and can't stop feeling empty
Tears run down my cheeks – everyone knows I'm hurting.
The things I found to relieve my pain became my greatest loves,
And now there is no one to comfort me.
My great loves have betrayed me,
My addictions have become my enemy.

My pain and addictions have enslaved me – and rule over me.
I am exhausted.
I have no place to go – nowhere to turn.
The people that once were important to me are gone.
I have no place to rest.
My pain and addictions pursued me, and have overtaken me,
In the midst of the worst moments of my life.

Nothing I do connects me to joy and life.
No one comes when I call for help – or even knows how to help me.
I've done everything I know how to do – and I still am empty, desolate and alone.
The people I thought were my friends hurt just as badly as I do.
There is no one I know who can help me.
Every good thing in me feels dead.

My addictions have become my master.
(Lamentations 1: 1-5, Author's Paraphrase).

I am happy to report that I have been in recovery from trauma and addictions for almost three decades. God has graciously helped me walk into the gift of recovery. I have found freedom from pain and addictions that I never dreamed possible. My heart and dreams are becoming ever more fully alive as I grow and mature in my relationship with Jesus – and with others who are empowered by joy.

One of the dreams that God has placed in my heart is for you.

My dream for you is that you would be able to walk fully into the freedom of recovery – and be empowered by joy to live from the heart and dreams that Jesus has placed within you. You and I have a destiny that is far beyond sobriety and freedom from pain. Our destiny is to become fully alive, connected in joy to God and others in relationships that are life giving. My dream for you is so big, that I believe you will discover the dreams that God has for you – and for others. You can become a source of help, healing and empowering joy for others like us who struggle.

This Restarting workbook is a part of my dream, and it is written for you.

Ed Khouri

WELCOME TO RESTARTING!
A REVOLUTION OF HOPE

You And I Are Created For Joy!
Joy-filled attachments to God and to others create joy in us, and help our brains learn to regulate emotion, pain and pleasure effectively. Synchronized relationships actually teach our brains to regulate dopamine (which helps us feel joy) and serotonin (which helps us quiet ourselves). In this way, we can learn to return to joy from negative emotions and develop secure attachments with God and others that are life giving. We feel alive, fulfilled – energized by the power of joy!

The Problem: A Lack Of Joyful Brain Training
Research strongly suggests that when our relationships with God and others are not joyful, the brain lacks the ability to effectively regulate emotions or consistently feel pleasure. We do not learn to live in joy, quiet ourselves when we are upset, or learn to handle negative emotions. We live in pain that our brains have not learned to regulate internally. This lack of joyful brain training affects every area of life from infancy – throughout adulthood.

Our capacity to connect with others in life giving relationships is one area greatly damaged by our lack of capacity for joy. Without a brain that is trained to attach to others in joy, our attachments with others seem to only perpetuate our pain. Relationships – that are designed by God to be a source of life and joy – become painful and sometimes toxic. This is highly painful and very traumatic – particularly when we didn't have much capacity to regulate negative emotions already. We tend to be locked in unending cycles of pain and broken relationships. Our pain feels unbearable.

Stuck in pain, and without joyful relationships with God and others, our brain lacks the skills and the attachments that are necessary to learn to regulate negative emotions and live in joy. The brain simply is unable to regulate our distress effectively. Lacking the joyful attachments with God and others that could help retrain it, our brain craves other attachments that might help medicate our pain. Addiction is the process by which the brain attaches to Behaviors, Events, Experiences, People and Substances (BEEPS) so that it can regulate emotion, increase pleasure and decrease pain.

Once our brain attaches itself to BEEPS, these attachments literally rewire our brain and alter the way it functions. In essence, BEEPS hijack the emotional control center of the brain responsible for attachment, emotional control and decision-making. When BEEPS are behind the wheel, they drive our lives and relationships to places of even greater pain.

The Search For Help
In desperation, we looked for help. We've tried support groups, counseling or treatment programs. We felt better, because caring people listened to our problems. "Talking things over" seemed to help – at least for a while, and we may have even changed our behaviors for a time. Inside, however, we were often left with a nagging sense that there was more to life than simply "not doing the wrong thing." Our relationships were still difficult, our joy capacity was low, and we struggled with difficult emotions.

Sometimes, we simply exchanged one problem behavior for another, or relapsed back into our addictions. We still needed BEEPS, because our brain was still unable to regulate our emotions, pain and pleasure effectively. We may have simply exchanged primary attachments to overtly destructive BEEPS such as alcohol or other illegal drugs to more hidden BEEPS such as work, perfection or food. We may have changed codependent relationships – but still felt empty, lost and frustrated on the inside. Our behaviors changed, but because

WELCOME TO RESTARTING!
A REVOLUTION OF HOPE

our brain had not learned to regulate emotions, pleasure and pain effectively, it still sought and found external attachments to medicate our distress. Our brain was still not sober.

Some of us turned to God and to the church for help. We longed for a deep sense of connection that could change our level of pain. Some of us were disappointed when the "quick fix" we hoped for did not come. We found that trying to do "the right things" to change, fit in and be accepted did not significantly change the pain and struggles we felt on the inside. Sometimes, we were frustrated because "God's people" did not seem to understand – or want to understand – our problems. When the spiritual or biblical advice they gave us did not bring about the promised "quick fix," some may even have blamed us for the failure and pulled away. We felt worse – not better.

At times, we were able to connect with others in God's family who genuinely cared for us, but simply did not know how to help us. They did not know that we were stuck because our brain had not learned to regulate our emotions effectively – and they did not know how to retrain our brain in joy. They cared – but caring was not enough. In our pain, we cried out, "God, is this the best you can do?" In our distress, we heard no answer – and concluded that God, and His people had no answers for us either. It was just one more experience in a long line of failures and disappointments.

Across The Line Of Despair
We tried secular and spiritual solutions, and still felt empty, frustrated, alone, and ashamed of our struggles and behaviors. In spite of sincere attempts to find help – and the sincere attempts of others to help us – we were unable to find lasting relief for our internal pain. Long-term solutions for our problem behaviors or addictions were beyond our reach. Even God seemed distant and without answers. We had no hope – but plenty of pain, shame and relationships that did not bring us joy. We had crossed the line of despair into hopelessness and rage.

When we cross the line of despair, many of us react differently. Since our brain has not been adequately trained to regulate our internal distress, our behaviors tend to be driven by pain and hopelessness. Some of us lash out at others, and take our frustrations out on the people closest to us. This not only hurts them – it hurts us as well. At times, despair may drive us further into self-destructive attachments with BEEPS. We may plunge back into our original addictions – or find new ones to numb our pain. Sometimes, we simply lapse into apathy and hopeless despair. We haven't been able to find solutions that work – and feel too hopeless to try anymore.

Restarting: A Revolution of Hope

We need a revolution of hope! The word revolution means, "a dramatic change in ideas or practice" (Microsoft Encarta Dictionary). We need a "dramatic change in our ideas and practice" about recovery that can bring us realistic hope of change. This is what Restarting is all about.

Restarting offers a solution-centered approach to recovery and change that is not focused on describing or talking about your problem in new or different ways. Restarting can help you lay a new foundation for change by helping you re-train your brain as you develop relationships with God and with others who are empowered by joy. In Restarting, you will learn simple joy and relationship building skills that help teach your brain to regulate emotions, pleasure and pain more effectively.

Restarting also is an opportunity to revolutionize your experience with God – and receive

WELCOME TO RESTARTING!
A REVOLUTION OF HOPE

healing from deep wounds and trauma from the past. Restarting will teach you simple exercises that help you experience the presence of Jesus in a way that is life giving and healing. Developing a conscious awareness of Jesus' presence keeps us in constant touch with the joy of One who is always glad to be with us.

Restarting also will give you the opportunity to become part of a community that is building joy together. You will find the support, joy and maturity you need to mature n the context of the life-giving relationships that can continue throughout the Thriving: Recover Your Life program. You will find yourself becoming more fully alive than you ever dreamed possible!

We Can Learn Practical Joy-Building, Relationship and Inner Healing Skills
Building joy in the context of secure, healthy relationships with God and others helps change our brain. As we learn to build joy and then experience quiet together with others, we are better able to regulate positive and negative emotions, pleasure and pain. As our capacity for joy grows, we are better able to respond to the stresses of life, without being overwhelmed.

Our increasing capacity for joy also allows us to form attachments and relationships with others that are secure. Our relationships become characterized by joy and mutual satisfaction. We are increasingly able to stay connected with each other when we are upset, and find that, instead of destroying our relationships, these challenges actually strengthen our bond with God and others. Joy is helping us choose attachments that are life-giving.

Our increasing capacity is also allowing us to begin to resolve painful life issues from our past. As we learn to experience the presence of Jesus, we find that He is able to bring hope and healing to the damaged and wounded areas of our hearts. He changes and heals us – from the inside out.

We Can Be Free From Attachments to BEEPS
As joy builds and our attachments and bonds with God and others become healthy, we find that unhealthy attachments to BEEPS become increasingly less important. Because our brain is being re-trained to regulate pain, pleasure and emotions in the context of joyful relationships with others, our brain is learning to handle our internal distress more effectively. It no longer needs BEEPS to medicate our pain. We find that we are increasingly able to live in the power of joy that gives us strength, transforms our lives, and helps us to grow into all that Jesus has created us to be.

Welcome to the Restarting Revolution
As you read this workbook, you will find that it is written for you – and for your Restarting facilitator. Feel free to take a look at the facilitator notes and chapter overviews that are located in the back of your workbook. You will also find that each chapter contains instructions for both you and your facilitator. By reading through each chapter, you will find out more about how your Restarting workbook is organized – and how your life can be transformed by the power of joy. Welcome to the revolution!

WELCOME TO RESTARTING!
HOW CAN I USE MY WORKBOOK?

You will need your workbook for every session of Restarting, so be sure to bring it with you to group. You will also need a pen or pencil to take notes or complete worksheets.

You will cover one chapter in your workbook each week. Each Restarting session includes a Restarting video as well as the exercises and material located in your workbook. Each chapter of your workbook contains:

- A complete list of everything that will be covered in your weekly Restarting group session.
- Instructions for each weekly exercise, along with facilitator notes.
- Teaching notes from your weekly Restarting video.
- Questions for further study.
- 12 Step questions for further study.
- Worksheets to help you complete Restarting group exercises.

To prepare for each Restarting session, it is a good idea to read through your chapter ahead of time. You will also find a more detailed overview of each chapter located in the Facilitator's Notes in the back of your workbook. Reading these overviews will help you better understand the purpose, goals and flow of each Restarting chapter and video.

During your Restarting group, you will have the opportunity to participate in many group exercises. Detailed instructions for each exercise are listed in each chapter, and your facilitator will go over these instructions with you. You are welcome to ask questions about anything that is unclear or that you do not understand. For some exercises, you will need worksheets that you will find in each chapter in which they are required.

Your workbook also contains teaching notes that accompany the video. Those of you who like to take notes will be relieved to find that every bit of text seen on the DVD is printed in outline form in your workbook. Each page of your workbook contains space for you to take notes.

You will also find it helpful to answer the questions at the end of each chapter. These questions are designed to function as study guides, and help you better understand and apply the most important concepts from each chapter and video. Because the questions are based on the weekly videos and group exercises, you will have to attend your Restarting group to best answer the questions. The teaching notes in your workbook will help you.

You do not have to complete the answers to these questions – they are for your growth and study only, and your regular weekly Restarting group will not discuss the questions. In some cases, your facilitator may offer Restarting study groups that will meet on other nights of the week to discuss the questions.

WELCOME TO RESTARTING!
GOD AND RESTARTING

From all credible reports, God is alive – and thriving! Because He has created us in His image, we have the same possibility: becoming fully alive in Him. This is the goal of Restarting - to be made fully alive in Him, flowing in the easy rhythm of the Spirit, and empowered to fulfill the unique purposes for which God has created us. Restarting, and the entire Thriving: Recover Your Life training flow begins and ends with this purpose.

Restarting teaches us that we are created in the image and likeness of God – and that means that we are created for joyful loving relationships with Him and others. In the context of joyful and loving relationships, our brains are trained according to their original design. By experiencing these joyful, synchronized relationships in the first two years of life, we are empowered to develop relationships with God and others that are secure and life giving. We are free to begin to discover our unique gifts and talents. The unique facets of our individual design, gifts and heart will be revealed when we connect in joyful relationships with God and others.

We develop an identity that is strong and healthy. We become rooted and grounded in love. The bonds we form with others – and with God – are joyful and life giving. Our group identity is strong and honoring to God. We are free to mature and grow according to the full capacity of our individual design. Our relationships with others are marked by healthy interdependence as together we are able to fulfill the purpose for which God's family is created.

We bring life wherever we go, and take the joy of secure attachments to places they've never been. We serve others and steward the life, resources and gifts we've been given. We can enjoy pleasure as God intended. We become family to those who are alone and care for their needs as the family of God. This is the vision of healthy relationships that Restarting is designed to help fulfill.

This is a work that begins and ends in the hope that is in Jesus.

Why are so many of us stuck in the pain of trauma and addiction? We want to be free – but we can't seem to make it past our past! To those of us who yearn for hope, Restarting offers you a revolutionary idea: You can be free!

What keeps us from flowing easily in joyful and quieting rhythms of grace? God has designed our brains so that they can be transformed – trained for joy, relationship and life until the day we die. We are never too old for relationship with Him and others that heal. Restarting offers participants an opportunity to encounter and experience the joyful and life giving relationships with God and others that can call our hearts back to life. In the context of a joyful, healing community, we can learn new skills that build our capacity for joy, learn to quiet ourselves and return to joy from negative emotions, and develop relationships with others that help us to heal. This is what God has known all along, we need to be connected with Him and with His family to thrive.

In addition, Restarting teaches us to perceive, experience and learn to live in the moment by moment awareness of the presence of Jesus. The Bible calls this "living by the Spirit." His life and presence bring fullness of joy, hope and healing. In Restarting, you will have the opportunity to learn simple prayer exercises that help you learn to experience the presence of Jesus. Because Jesus is Lord of All – past, present and future – He can heal our painful wounds from the past.

Restarting is about beginning a new life in recovery that is full of hope and freedom. If you are suffering from the painful experience of trauma, or unhealthy attachments to Behaviors, Events, Experiences, People or Substances – Restarting offers you a new opportunity to walk more fully into your destiny. As your heart is healing, you will find that you are becoming more fully alive. You are awakening to the possibilities of the dreams that God has dreamed for you.

RESTARTING GROUP
GROUND RULES

Please read these important rules before attending your first Restarting group. These rules are intended to make Restarting a safe, healthy and healing experience for all. If you have questions about any of them, please ask your facilitator.

- Confidentiality is a fundamental group rule. Confidentiality means that what an individual participant in a Restarting group shares should never be repeated by another participant outside of group at any time – without explicit permission in advance. Please understand that your facilitator may have a legal obligation to report to the proper authorities:
  - A person is in immediate danger of hurting themselves, others or the property of others.
  - Child abuse or abuse of the elderly.
- Exercises that help participants build joyful bonds together are powerful. For this reason, all small group exercises must be done in groups of 3-5 people. Forming "couple bonds" with others you meet in Restarting is a good recipe for disaster.
- Participation in all group exercises is encouraged – but voluntary.
- Feedback offered in small group exercises should be consistent with the instructions given with that exercise.
- Supportive active listening is always appropriate. Personal advice and criticism are not.
- Restarting participants should arrive for group without being intoxicated or under the influence of psychoactive drugs. Intoxication or the use of mind-altering BEEPS keeps your brain from being able to learn and train. If you are under the influence you may be referred to a Thriving crisis group (if available) or invited to return the following week when sober.
- Threats, intimidation or violence of any kind will result in immediate dismissal from group.

Since one of your facilitator's tasks is to help keep you and your group safe, they will have to respond appropriately to violations of these group ground rules. In almost all cases, you and your facilitator can resolve the issue. In very few cases, you may not be able to return to Restarting until the problem has been addressed and resolved in a way that is appropriate – and helps keep you and your group safe.

RESTARTING
WORKBOOK

FOR USE WITH THE RESTARTING DVD SERIES
TWELVE WEEKS COURSE WORKBOOK

1 TRAIN YOUR BRAIN FOR A CHANGE
HOW IS THE BRAIN ORGANIZED? WHAT DOES IT NEED?

OPEN THE GROUP

- Ask for a volunteer to open the group in prayer.

APPRECIATION EXERCISE: *10-15 Minutes*

Facilitator Note: This joy and capacity building exercise asks participants to identify a person that they appreciate, and a time in which they felt especially grateful to be with them.

Several important components of joy and capacity building exercises are introduced in this exercise.

First, as volunteers share, they are asked to maintain appropriate eye contact with other group members. Learning to maintain appropriate eye contact is an important relationship building skill that helps retrain the brain. Joy is communicated non-verbally through eye contact when others are "glad to be with us." The experience of others "being glad to be with us" helps build joy, and is an essential part of Restarting exercises. It is helpful to remind participants that while eye contact is important, this is not a staring contest!

Second, as volunteers share about the person and moment they appreciate, they are encouraged to describe the specific emotions and body sensations they felt during the experience. Sharing the specific experience, and the accompanying emotions and body sensations helps activate the right orbital prefrontal cortex of the brain. Activation of this region of the brain is essential for learning.

Next, it is important to remind participants that all small group exercises must be done in groups of 3-5 people. This helps participants remain safe as they are building joyful bonds that help retrain the brain.

Finally, please note that sharing in small group is strongly encouraged, but is not required. It is also important to remind participants that they can support each other through active listening and appropriate eye contact. Listen – but please do not offer comments, criticism or advice in response to what others have shared.

YOUR NOTES

1. Break into small groups of 3-5 people.

2. Your facilitator will explain that this exercise has several purposes:
   a. This exercise helps build joy and relationship skills.
   b. This exercise helps activate the right orbital prefrontal cortex of your brain. Activation of this area of the brain is essential for learning.

3. Your facilitator will ask you to think about a person that you appreciate and a time you felt especially grateful to be with that person.

4. Your facilitator will share with you about his or her special person for one minute.

TRAIN YOUR BRAIN FOR A CHANGE
HOW IS THE BRAIN ORGANIZED? WHAT DOES IT NEED?

YOUR NOTES

As your facilitator shares, he/she will:
a. Maintain eye contact while sharing.
b. Identify the person he/she appreciates, and describe a moment when he/she was especially grateful to be with them.
c. Describe the emotions he/she felt while he/she was with them.
d. Describe what his/her body felt like when he/she was with them.

5. Your facilitator will remind you of a few simple guidelines for this exercise:
   a. All Restarting exercises are done in groups of 3-5 people.
   b. Sharing in small group is strongly encouraged, but is not required.
   c. Support each other through active listening and appropriate eye contact.
   d. Please do not offer comments, criticism or advice in response to what others have shared.

6. Your facilitator will ask volunteers to each share for one minute about the person they appreciate. As you share, be sure to:
   a. Maintain appropriate eye contact while sharing. Remember, this exercise is joy-building – not a staring contest!
   b. Identify the person you appreciate, and describe a moment when you were especially grateful to be with them.
   c. Describe what emotions you felt while you were with them.
   d. Describe what your body felt like when you were with them.

7. When each group is finished, your facilitator may ask volunteers to share with the entire group how they felt before and after the exercise. Use one or two words to describe your feelings.

TODAY'S LESSON: How is the Brain Organized? What Does It Need?

Facilitator Notes: Play Session One on the Restarting DVD.
- Ask the class to follow along in their workbooks, and take notes as needed.

CLASS NOTES: How is the Brain Organized? What Does it Need?

How are we created?
- Then God said, "Let Us make man in Our image, according to Our likeness… Then God saw everything that He had made, and indeed it was very good.

  Genesis 1:26, 31. NKJV.

  Let us: God is relational!
  Make man in our image: created by God in his image and his likeness - relational.
  It was very good: God was really happy with the way we turned out.
- We function according to our original design – like God when we are in relationship with Him and with each other.

We are designed so that our brain functions best when it is in secure relationships!
- I will praise You, for I am fearfully and wonderfully made; Marvelous are your works, and that my soul knows very well. Psalm 139:14, NKJV.

The brain is created with 2 hemispheres
- The 2 hemispheres are different.
- They are designed to work together.
- The brain works best when each side is healthy and they are synchronized together.

TRAIN YOUR BRAIN FOR A CHANGE
HOW IS THE BRAIN ORGANIZED? WHAT DOES IT NEED?

YOUR NOTES

Left and right
- Left side: naming and explaining
- Right side: knowing and experiencing

The left hemisphere
- A place of words and language
- A place of stories
- A place of descriptions
- A place of explanations, logic and reasoning
- Very resistant to change
- Persists in the face of contrary evidence
- Open to change only when the right hemisphere is "upset"

The right hemisphere
- Non-verbal
- Imagistic
- Prosodic (voice tone)
- Executive control system of the brain
- Contains a four-level emotional brain structure
- Dominant for emotions and body
- Synchronizes and notices "everything"
- Decides when the left hemisphere can change beliefs

In the right brain: a four level control center
- *Level One:*
  - Attachment
  - Thalamus and basal ganglia, help regulate dopamine
- *Level Two:*
  - The guardshack: life is good, bad or scary
  - The amygdala: helps regulate adrenaline
- *Level Three:*
  - Synchronization
  - The cingulate cortex: helps regulate serotonin
  - Helps resolve negative emotions
- *Level Four:*
  - Identity
  - The right orbital prefrontal cortex
  - Helps me focus my attention, and answer the question "Who am I?"

Relationships are the building blocks for healthy brains
- The right brain's emotional control center starts developing from birth.
- Level 1 attachment is the foundation for this growth.
- A healthy control center allows the right brain and the later developing left brain to be well synchronized and have healthy connections.
- Relationships are the foundation for the development and integration of the entire brain!

Dr. Allan Schore
- Affect Regulation and Origin of the Self
- Affect Regulation and the Repair of the Self
- Affect Dysregulation and Disorders of the Self

TRAIN YOUR BRAIN FOR A CHANGE
HOW IS THE BRAIN ORGANIZED? WHAT DOES IT NEED?

For healthy development, the brain needs joyful relationships.

Joy means relationships!

Joy means: we are glad to be together. Someone is glad to be with me!

Right-hemisphere to right-hemisphere communication
- Right brain > left face > left side of retinas > right brain
- Six complete cycles of communication every second
- Synchronized brain chemistry
- Matched brain structure growth
- Authentic, truthful, rapid communication
- Emotions are AMPLIFIED each cycle
- Subjectively experienced as produced by the "other"

Climbing Joy Mountain: capacity

When our joy capacity is low, life is painful.
- The deepest level of pain is attachment pain at level 1 of the control center.

Medicate to regulate

BEEPS
- BEEPS are attachments to Behaviors, Events, Experiences, People or Substances that are used to regulate emotions, increase pleasure or decrease pain.

BEEPS
- Attachments to BEEPS help us medicate – to artificially regulate – positive and negative emotions as well as pain.

BEEPS
- Attachments to BEEPS take the place of secure attachments to God and significant others.

BEEPS
- There are many different types of BEEPS.
- Behaviors: Work
- Events: Thrill Seeking
- Experiences: Sex
- People: Relationships
- Substances: Alcohol

Thriving and the Twelve Steps
- Since the 1930's the Twelve Steps and self-help support groups have helped millions of men and women around the world find hope and sobriety.
- Thriving, through the advances in research made in "The Decade of the Brain," is a program designed to help participants become healthy, whole, sober and mature.
- Thriving teaches participants the joy and relationship building skills that the brain needs to heal – and remain sober – through the development of secure, healthy attachments with God and others in a mature, life-giving community.

TRAIN YOUR BRAIN FOR A CHANGE
HOW IS THE BRAIN ORGANIZED? WHAT DOES IT NEED?

YOUR NOTES

BEEPS promise relief but make life unmanageable
- Step 1: We admitted we were powerless over BEEPS – that our lives had become unmanageable.

BEEPS attachments are sub-cortical
- BEEPS affect the attachment center of the brain.
- The brain is designed so that dopamine and endogenous opiates are released when people are "glad to be with us."
- This is the neurochemistry of joy!

BEEPS fool the attachment center
- BEEPS also trigger the release of dopamine and stimulate the pleasure center of the brain.
- BEEPS mimic genuine joyful relationships.
- In this way, the attachment center is fooled into attaching to BEEPS to regulate every single emotion, pleasure and pain.

BEEPS hijack the attachment center
- The attachment center learns to rely on BEEPS – and not relationships with God and others that produce joy.
- In this way, BEEPS hijack the attachment center.
- When BEEPS take over, life becomes unmanageable – we end up in places we never wanted to go.

Recovering our life means becoming connected in joyful relationships with God and with other people.

And that is why we need joy & relationships!

EXERCISE: The Father Wound Video Discussion: *20-25 Minutes*
After watching Rocky in the "Father Wound Video"

Facilitator Notes: This exercise provides participants the chance to share their impressions of Rocky's experience in the Father Wound video. Volunteers may share their impressions by answering a series of questions about the video. Because this video can be painful for participants who have experienced father wounds, these questions ask participants to focus their attention on:
- The dramatic change that occurred in Rocky during the prayer ministry session and the follow-up interview.
- Any emotions experienced while watching the video.
- Why it was important for Rocky to experience Jesus "being glad to be with him" at a very painful moment of life.
- What happened to Rocky's weight and attachment to food.
- The potential importance of this process for our own healing from trauma and attachments to BEEPS.

Volunteers are encouraged to stay relational with each other as they share by maintaining appropriate eye contact. It is also important to remind them that they can support each other by active listening. Please do not give advice or offer criticism or corrective comments about what others have shared.

TRAIN YOUR BRAIN FOR A CHANGE
HOW IS THE BRAIN ORGANIZED? WHAT DOES IT NEED?

YOUR NOTES

1. Break into groups of 3-5 people.

2. Volunteers may share answers to the following questions about the video:
   a. What was your impression of how different Rocky looked during the session and then at follow-up?
   b. What was the difference in Rocky's life after the session with Dr. Lehman?
   c. How did you feel when you watched Rocky's video?
   d. In the video, Rocky experienced Jesus being "glad to be with him" at a very painful moment of his life. Why was this important for Rocky?
   e. What happened to Rocky's attachment to food?
   f. Do you think this healing process can be important for our own recovery from trauma and attachments to BEEPS?

3. Your facilitator will remind you to:
   a. Stay relational by making appropriate eye contact as you share.
   b. Support each other by actively listening as others share.
   c. Please do not give advice or offer criticism or corrective comments about what others have shared.

4. Your facilitator will help you by keeping track of time.

5. Following the small group sharing, your facilitator may ask volunteers to share their insights and responses with the entire group. (Approximately 10 minutes.)

CLOSE THE GROUP WITH PRAYER

TRAIN YOUR BRAIN FOR A CHANGE
HOW IS THE BRAIN ORGANIZED? WHAT DOES IT NEED?

QUESTIONS FOR FURTHER DISCUSSION OR FOLLOW-UP

1. How did God create our brains, and why do we need relationships?
2. What are the dominant functions of the *left hemisphere* of the brain?
3. What are the dominant functions of the *right hemisphere* of the brain?
4. Where is the *four level control center* located, and why is it important?
5. What does the brain need for healthy development?
6. What is joy?
7. Why is it important to build increasing joy capacity?
8. What happens when our joy capacity is low?
9. What are BEEPS, and why are they important?
10. Did you recognize attachments to BEEPS in your own life?
11. Did you recognize attachments to BEEPS in the lives of important people in your life, such as family members and friends?
12. How do BEEPS hijack the attachment center of my brain, and why do BEEPS make my life unmanageable?
13. What do I need to recover my life?

TRAIN YOUR BRAIN FOR A CHANGE
HOW IS THE BRAIN ORGANIZED? WHAT DOES IT NEED?

OPTIONAL 12 STEP QUESTIONS

1. What was the first BEEPS you ever used?

2. What other BEEPS have you used?

3. What are your BEEPS attachments now?

4. What happened the first time you used BEEPS? What did you feel like before and after?

5. What happened the last time you used BEEPS?

6. How have your attachments to BEEPS caused you problems in relationships? Have you ever damaged or lost a relationship through your attachments to BEEPS? Think about relationships with your parents, brothers & sisters, spouse, children, family and close friends.

7. Have your attachments with BEEPS ever caused you problems with work?
Have you ever lost a job or gotten in trouble for use of BEEPS at work? Think about issues like being late for work or missing work because of BEEPS use. Have you ever used BEEPS on the job – or at lunch?

8. Have your attachments to BEEPS ever gotten you in legal trouble?

9. How have attachments to BEEPS impacted your physical health?

10. Have you lost things you valued as a result of your attachments to BEEPS? Think about things like: relationships, jobs, health, houses, cars, values, dignity and respect.

11. How have your attachments to BEEPS affected the way you feel about yourself? How do you feel when you think about how BEEPS have affected your life and relationships?

12. On a scale of 1 (lowest) – 10 (highest), describe how painful BEEPS attachments have been in your life.

13. Have you ever tried to give up an attachment to BEEPS? What happened?

14. Do you think that BEEPS have hijacked part of your life?

15. What do the words powerless and unmanageability mean to you?

2 THE 2 SKILLS YOUR BRAIN CAN'T LIVE WITHOUT
THE RHYTHMS OF JOY AND QUIET

OPEN THE GROUP

- Ask for a volunteer to open the group in prayer.

APPRECIATION EXERCISE: *5 Minutes*

Facilitator Note: This is a joy and capacity building exercise that helps prepare participants for this week's lesson. In this exercise, participants share about an experience from the past week in which they felt appreciation for someone or something.

As you recall from last week's lesson, this appreciation exercise helps train the brain in several ways. When volunteers maintain appropriate eye contact with others as they share, they are building joyful capacity and bonds – and training the emotional control center in the brain's right hemisphere. In addition, by sharing the specific emotions and body sensations that accompanied the appreciation experience, participants are activating the right orbital prefrontal cortex of the brain. Activation of this region of the brain is essential for learning.

Since this is only the second week of Restarting, it is helpful to remind participants of the following:
- Sharing in small group is strongly encouraged, but is not required.
- Support each other through active listening and appropriate eye contact.
- Please do not offer comments, criticism or advice in response to what others have shared.

1. Break into small groups of 3-5 people.

2. Your facilitator will explain that this exercise has several purposes.
   a. This exercise helps build joy and relationship skills.
   b. This exercise helps activate the right orbital prefrontal cortex of your brain. Activation of this area of the brain is essential for learning.

3. Your facilitator will ask you to think about an experience in the past week in which you felt appreciation for someone or something.

4. Your facilitator will take one minute to share his/her appreciation moment with you. He/she will:
   a. Maintain eye contact while sharing.
   b. Describe the appreciation experience, person or moment.
   c. Describe what emotions they felt during that experience.
   d. Describe what their body felt like during that experience.

5. Your facilitator will remind you of a few simple guidelines for this exercise:
   a. Sharing in small group is strongly encouraged, but is not required.
   b. Support each other through active listening and appropriate eye contact.
   c. Please do not offer comments, criticism or advice in response to what others have shared.

YOUR NOTES

24 | **Thriving:** Recover Your Life, *Session Two*

THE 2 SKILLS YOUR BRAIN CAN'T LIVE WITHOUT
THE RHYTHMS OF JOY AND QUIET

YOUR NOTES

6. Your facilitator will ask volunteers to each share for one minute about the person or moment that they appreciate. As you share, remember to:
   a. Maintain appropriate eye contact while sharing. Remember, this is a joy building exercise – not a staring contest!
   b. Describe person or experience you appreciate.
   c. Describe what emotions you felt during that experience.
   d. Describe what your body felt like during that experience.

7. When each group is finished, your facilitator may ask volunteers to share with the entire group how they felt before and after the exercise. Volunteers should use one or two words to describe their feelings.

EXERCISE: LEARN TO RELAX AND BREATHE DEEPLY *10 Minutes.*

Facilitator Note: This exercise involves progressive muscle relaxation. It is designed to help participants learn to breathe deeply and relax their body. They are also sharing "quiet together."

Please make sure that you give the following instruction before leading this exercise. "If you are concerned about your physical ability to do this exercise, or if you have any spine, bone or muscle injury, weakness or problem, please consult with your doctor before you attempt this exercise. The breathing portions of this exercise may be done while seated, and can be practiced without the muscle relaxation segments of this exercise."

1. Before beginning this exercise, your facilitator will advise you that:
   a. If you are concerned about your physical ability to do this exercise, or if you have any spine, bone or muscle injury, weakness or problem, please consult with your doctor before attempting this exercise.
   b. The breathing portions of this exercise may be done while seated, and can be practiced without the muscle relaxation segments of this exercise.

2. Please follow your facilitator's instructions as you do this exercise.

3. Stand up, and make sure that you have 3-4 feet of clear space around you.

4. Imagine that you are a marionette – a puppet – with a string running from the base of your spine to the top of your head. Imagine that the string is gently pulled upwards and your back, neck and head are perfectly aligned. Your head is at rest and comfortably settled in line with your back and spine. You are looking forward, and your head is settled in comfortably.

5. Bend your knees slightly. Your are standing still in a comfortable position.

6. Place your hand over your stomach.

7. Take such a deep breath that you feel your stomach expand as you breathe. Follow your facilitator's instructions as you breathe deeply for a few moments.
   a. When we are stressed, we tend to take rapid shallow breaths. By learning deep breathing exercises and paying attention to what our bodies are doing, we make sure our brain is receiving enough oxygen, and we are activating the

THE 2 SKILLS YOUR BRAIN CAN'T LIVE WITHOUT
THE RHYTHMS OF JOY AND QUIET

> **YOUR NOTES**

     right orbital prefrontal cortex of our brain. Both of these are needed for learning.
- b. Practicing deep breathing exercises can also help us think through our options when we are distressed, and avoid making poor decisions made in hasty reactions to stress.

8. Follow your facilitator's instructions as you learn to relax your face, shoulders, arms, hands, legs, and feet. You will alternately tighten and then loosen the muscles in these areas as you follow your facilitator's directions.
   - a. You may choose to remain standing, sit, or lay down on the floor during this segment of the exercise.

9. Continue to breathe deeply as your body is relaxing.

10. Return to your seats when the exercise is complete and it is time to start the Week 2 Video.

TODAY'S LESSON: The 2 Skills Your Brain Can't Live Without
The Rhythms of Joy and Quiet

Facilitator Note: Play Session Two on the Restarting DVD.
- Ask the class to follow along in their workbooks, and take notes as needed.

CLASS NOTES: The Rhythms of Joy and Quiet

A quick review:
- Last week, we learned that we are created so that our brain functions best when it is in secure relationships.

Left and right sides of the brain
- Left Side: Naming and Explaining
- Right Side: Knowing and Experiencing

In the right brain: a four level control center
- *Level One:*
  - Attachment
  - Thalamus and basal ganglia, help regulate dopamine
- *Level Two:*
  - The guardshack: life is good, bad or scary
  - The amygdala: helps regulate adrenaline
- *Level Three:*
  - Synchronization
  - The cingulate cortex: helps regulate serotonin
  - Helps resolve negative emotions
- *Level Four:*
  - Identity
  - The right orbital prefrontal cortex
  - Helps me focus my attention, and answer the question "Who am I?"

Creation reflects rhythms of joy and quiet
- Then God said, "Let there be lights in the firmament of the heavens to divide the day from the night; and let them be for signs and seasons, and for days and years;

THE 2 SKILLS YOUR BRAIN CAN'T LIVE WITHOUT
THE RHYTHMS OF JOY AND QUIET

and let them be for lights in the firmament of the heavens to give light on the earth"; and it was so....And God saw that it was good. Genesis 1: 14-15, 18. NKJV.

- We are also creatures of rhythm.

When we move easily from rhythms of joy into rhythms of quiet in relationships:
- Our brain works best.
- How do we learn the rhythms of joy and quiet?
- We learn these rhythms in relationships!

We are created for joy
- Joy is our natural state
- Joy creates our identity
- Joy is the basis for bonding
- Joy gives us our strength

Joy is why Jesus spoke to us
- "These things I have spoken to you, that my joy may be in you, and that your joy may be full." John 15:11, RSV.

How do we build joy?

Joy means relationships

Joy means: we are glad to be together. Someone is glad to be with me!

Attachment, joy and the senses: myelination of the sensory regions
- 0-6 weeks
    - Taste
    - Temperature regulation
    - Smell
- 6-12 weeks touch
- 2-12 months visual
- 12-24 months voice tone

Joy smiles synchronize mother and child from 2 – 12 months.

Right-hemisphere to right-hemisphere communication
- Right brain > left face > left side of retinas > right brain
- Six complete cycles of communication every second
- Synchronized brain chemistry
- Matched brain structure growth
- Authentic, truthful, rapid communication
- Emotions are AMPLIFIED each cycle
- Subjectively experienced as produced by the "other"

Climbing Joy Mountain: capacity
- Learning to build joy and increase capacity are tasks for the first year of life.

Before visual cortex myelination (6 weeks)
- The "dead shark" stare
- Too young for right-hemisphere to right-hemisphere communication.
- No joy amplification yet!

3 months - visual cortex ready for joy amplification (right hemisphere)

THE 2 SKILLS YOUR BRAIN CAN'T LIVE WITHOUT
THE RHYTHMS OF JOY AND QUIET

Smile for the camera

Smile for joy

Low and high joy levels
- Can you find the baby in high joy?
- Can you find the baby in low joy?
- Who is "smiling for the camera?"

How do we learn rhythms of quiet together?

We are created for quiet together
- Quiet Together is our natural state
- Quiet Together creates our identity
- Quiet Together is the basis for bonding
- Quiet Together gives us our strength

Quiet together means:
- We are not alone.
- We can rest.
- I can still and quiet myself.
- I am undisturbed – even in the presence of my enemies, for someone is with me.

Disruption of "quiet together time" is the strongest predictor of developing a mental illness.
- SPECT Scan of a brain in depression from Dr. Daniel Amen.
- The cingulate cortex is over-active.

***Healing The Hardware of the Soul* by Dr. Daniel Amen.**
- Very practical lists and steps to help your brain work better and correct problems that produce emotional symptoms.
- Good brain scans!
- Visit www.amenclinic.com or www.brainplace.com for more information and other brain scans.

Mom and baby building joy and then sharing quiet together
- Mom and baby build joy together.
- Baby looks up and left when rest is needed.
- Mom synchronizes with baby.
- Baby and mom then share "Quiet Together"
- Field and Fogel, 1982 in "Origin of the Self" by Dr. Alan Schore, p 86.

Visual experiences and socio-emotional development
- *Unsynchronized Mother and Baby*
  - Mom is not synchronized with the baby's emotional state, and does not respond appropriately to the baby's state of emotional arousal.
  - Baby is overwhelmed
  - There is no sharing of "Quiet Together."
- *Synchronized Mother and Baby*
  - Mom is synchronized, and responds appropriately to the baby's state of emotional arousal.
  - Baby and mom share joy together
  - Baby and mom share "Quiet Together."
- This is from the work of Dr. Allan Schore.

THE 2 SKILLS YOUR BRAIN CAN'T LIVE WITHOUT
THE RHYTHMS OF JOY AND QUIET

We learn to synch – or sink!

Mom and baby building joy and then sharing quiet together
- "Mother Core" synchronization
- Mom and baby synchronize and build joy together.
- Baby looks up and left when rest is needed.
- Mom would then synchronize with the baby, and they would then share "Quiet Together."
- Beebe and Lachman, 1988 in "Affect Regulation and Origin of the Self" by Dr. Allan Schore, p 81.

Photos of mom and baby sharing joy and synchronizing together
- Good mother (both low)
- Good mother (both medium)
- Just before disconnect to rest
- This is where they would share "Quiet Together" time.

We are creatures of rhythm
- Rhythmic change is our natural state.
- Rhythmic change creates our identity.
- Rhythmic change is the basis for bonding.
- Rhythmic change gives us our strength.

We learn to synch – or sink!

When our joy capacity is low, and we can't quiet ourselves, life is very painful
- We experience trauma when our level of pain exceeds our level of joy.
- Pervasive fear is pain at level 2 of the emotional control center.

Medicate to Regulate

BEEPS
- BEEPS are attachments to Behaviors, Events, Experiences, People or Substances that are used to regulate emotions, increase pleasure or decrease pain.

BEEPS
- Attachments to BEEPS help us medicate – to artificially regulate – positive and negative emotions as well as pain.

BEEPS
- Attachments to BEEPS take the place of secure attachments to God and significant others.

BEEPS
- There are many different types of BEEPS. Examples can include:
- Behaviors: Work
- Events: Thrill Seeking
- Experiences: Sex
- People: Relationships
- Substances: Alcohol

Wired to BEEPS
- Step 1: We admitted we were powerless over BEEPS - that our lives had become unmanageable.

THE 2 SKILLS YOUR BRAIN CAN'T LIVE WITHOUT
THE RHYTHMS OF JOY AND QUIET

YOUR NOTES

- Using BEEPS to regulate emotions, pleasure and pain wires the brain to BEEPS.

The longer beeps are used, the stronger the connection becomes

Losing control
- Eventually, the response between unwanted emotions and pain is so strong, that the response is automatic.

BEEPS wiring leaves us powerless and life is unmanageable

Rhythms of joy and quiet rewire the brain to connect with God and others, and disconnect from BEEPS.

EXERCISE: The Mother Wound Video Discussion: *20-25 Minutes*
After watching Eileen in the "Mother Wound Video"

> **Facilitator Note:** This exercise provides participants the chance to share their impressions of Eileen's experience in the Mother Wound video. Volunteers may share their impressions by answering a series of questions about the video. Because this video can be painful for participants who have experienced mother wounds, these questions ask participants to focus their attention on:
> - The dramatic change that occurred in Eileen's life and appearance between the prayer ministry session and the follow-up interview.
> - Any emotions experienced while watching Eileen decide to come to Jesus,
> - The importance of Eileen's decision to come to Jesus.
> - Eileen's experience and description of Jesus' smile.
> - Eileen's attachment to ice cream and comfort eating.
> - The potential importance of this process for our own healing from trauma and attachments to BEEPS.
>
> Volunteers are encouraged to stay relational with each other as they share by maintaining appropriate eye contact. It is also important to remind them that they can support each other by active listening. Please do not give advice or offer criticism or corrective comments about what others have shared.

1. Break into groups of 3-5 people.

2. Volunteers may share answers to the following questions about the video:
   a. Did you notice a difference in Eileen's appearance between the prayer session and the follow-up?
   b. What was the difference in Eileen's life after the session with Dr. Lehman?
   c. How did you feel when you watched Eileen struggling with her decision to come to Jesus?
   d. Why was it important for Eileen to make a decision to go to Jesus? Why did Jesus wait for her to come to Him?

THE 2 SKILLS YOUR BRAIN CAN'T LIVE WITHOUT
THE RHYTHMS OF JOY AND QUIET

YOUR NOTES

    e. In the video, Eileen refers to Jesus' smile. After what we've learned in this week's lesson, why is that important?

    f. What happened to Eileen's "comfort eating" and her attachment with ice cream?

    g. What do you think would happen if you could learn to experience the presence of Jesus in the painful places of your own life?

3. Your facilitator will remind you to:
   a. Stay relational by making appropriate eye contact as you share.
   b. Support each other by actively listening as others share.
   c. Please do not give advice or offer criticism or corrective comments about what others have shared.

4. Your facilitator will help you by keeping track of time.

5. Following the small group sharing, your facilitator may ask volunteers to share their insights and responses with the entire group. (Approx 10 minutes).

CLOSE THE GROUP WITH PRAYER

THE 2 SKILLS YOUR BRAIN CAN'T LIVE WITHOUT
THE RHYTHMS OF JOY AND QUIET

QUESTIONS FOR FURTHER DISCUSSION OR FOLLOW-UP

1. How do we learn the rhythms of joy and quiet?

2. Why did Jesus say that joy was important?

3. What is the primary way that moms and babies bond from 2-12 months?

4. Why is quiet together important for the brain?

5. What do rhythms of joy and quiet teach us?

6. Who built joy and quiet together time with you when you were a child?

7. How do you feel when you make eye contact with family and close friends? Why?

8. What are the messages you learned about eye contact from your family?

9. Who builds joy with you?

10. Are you able to effectively quiet and calm yourself when you are upset? What do you need to learn to more effectively quiet yourself?

11. Do you feel like your level of pain often exceeds your level of joy? How long? Have you felt that your level of joy was not high enough to handle the pain in your life?

12. What happens when your level of joy is overwhelmed by pain?

13. Have you ever used BEEPS to avoid feelings that you didn't like?

14. What BEEPS did you use to relieve those feelings?

15. What happens when you do not use BEEPS to medicate those feelings?

16. Have you ever decided that you didn't want to use BEEPS – but felt so overwhelmed that you used BEEPS anyway?

THE 2 SKILLS YOUR BRAIN CAN'T LIVE WITHOUT
THE RHYTHMS OF JOY AND QUIET

OPTIONAL 12 STEP QUESTIONS

1. Do you think that you've lost control of your attachments to BEEPS? Why?

2. Can you remember a time when you felt like you were able to control your use of BEEPS? Do you still feel that way now?

3. Did you ever use BEEPS when you did not plan on it? What happened?

4. Have you ever felt guilty and ashamed because of your use of BEEPS?

5. Have you ever experienced weight loss or gain that is a direct result of your use of BEEPS? Describe your experience.

6. Have BEEPS ever resulted in the loss of a relationship that was important to you? Describe your experience.

7. Have you ever spent money on BEEPS that you knew should have been spent on other people or things? What happened?

8. Have you ever promised others that you would cut back or stop using BEEPS? Who did you promise, and what happened? Were you able to fulfill your promise?

9. Have people close to you ever told you that they thought BEEPS were a problem for you? Who were they, and how did you respond?

10. Has your use of BEEPS ever bothered you?

11. Think about the times when you have used BEEPS. What do you usually feel like just before you use BEEPS?

12. Have you ever felt angry, sad, hopeless, afraid, disgusted or ashamed– and used BEEPS to stop the pain?

13. Have you ever used BEEPS to calm down?

14. Do you think that BEEPS help you medicate unwanted feelings?

15. Can you imagine living without BEEPS? Describe what you think your life might be like – and feel like – without BEEPS.

16. What does powerlessness mean to you?

17. What do you think you need to start dealing with the powerlessness and unmanageability that are a part of BEEPS?

3 CALMING OUR PAINFUL EMOTIONS
RETURNING TO JOY, PART 1: SYNCHRONIZATION & NEGATIVE EMOTIONS

OPEN THE GROUP

- Ask for a volunteer to open the group in prayer.

SYNCHRONIZED WALKING: *20 Minutes*

Facilitator Note: This activity will require enough room for participants to walk around the room in groups of 3. You may need to clear space by moving chairs or tables so that everyone has enough room.

This exercise illustrates the concept of "synchronization," which is an important component of this week's lesson. We learn to return to joy from negative emotions when others who are empowered by joy are willing to share our distress and stay connected with us when we feel a negative emotion. This process of emotional synchronization trains our brain to return to joy from distressing negative emotions.

In this synchronized walking exercise, participants learn to synchronize with each other by matching stride, gait and physical mannerisms as they walk together in groups of 3. This simple exercise provides a visible illustration of the concept of synchronization – and is also a lot of fun! After participants learn to synchronize while walking normally, it is time to try advanced synchronizing skills – with silly walks!

1. Your facilitator will introduce you to the concept of "synchronization," that is one of this week's topics. Synchronized walking is a good way to have fun and introduce this concept.

2. Stand up and form small groups of 3 people.

3. Follow your facilitator's instructions – as they help you and your groups line up.
   a. Each person in a group of 3 should stand side-by-side.
   b. All the small groups should form a circle around the room with plenty of space between them.

4. Your facilitator will signal the groups to start walking in a circle around the room.

5. The person in the middle of each small group walks normally. The others in their small group synchronize with the person in the middle by copying their walk and movements.

6. After the groups are synchronizing fairly well, your facilitator will let the groups know that the person in the middle of each small group can change their walk (silly walks are encouraged) and have their partners continue to synchronize with them. This can be lots of fun!

7. After 2 minutes, your facilitator will signal you that it is time to switch places. The person in the middle moves to the outside, and a new person moves into the middle. The entire exercise repeats.

YOUR NOTES

CALMING OUR PAINFUL EMOTIONS
RETURNING TO JOY, PART 1: SYNCHRONIZATION & NEGATIVE EMOTIONS

YOUR NOTES

8. After 2 minutes, your facilitator will signal you that it is time to switch places. The person who has not yet had a turn in the middle moves to the middle. The exercise repeats.

9. After 2 minutes, your facilitator will ask everyone to return to their seats, but remain together in groups of 3.

10. Your facilitator will ask each group to take 5 minutes and share what it felt like to synchronize together.

11. At the end of 5 minutes, your facilitator may ask volunteers to share their experience with synchronized walking with the entire group.

TODAY'S LESSON: Returning to Joy, Part One:
Synchronization and Negative Emotions.

Facilitator Note: Play Session Three on the Restarting DVD.
- Ask the class to follow along in their workbooks, and take notes as needed.
- There is a group exercise during the video. When it is time for the exercise, stop the video and follow the instructions that are listed in the Class Notes.

CLASS NOTES: Returning to Joy, Part 1

A quick review:
- Last week, we learned that we are created so that our brain functions best when it is in secure relationships.

Left and right sides of the brain
- Left side: naming and explaining
- Right side: knowing and experiencing

In the right brain: a four level control center
- Level One:
  - Attachment
  - Thalamus and basal ganglia, help regulate dopamine
- Level Two:
  - The guardshack: life is good, bad or scary
  - The amygdala: helps regulate adrenaline
- Level Three:
  - Synchronization
  - The cingulate cortex: helps regulate serotonin
  - Helps resolve negative emotions
- Level Four:
  - Identity
  - The right orbital prefrontal cortex
  - Helps me focus my attention, and answer the question "Who am I?"

Joy means relationships

CALMING OUR PAINFUL EMOTIONS
RETURNING TO JOY, PART 1: SYNCHRONIZATION & NEGATIVE EMOTIONS

Joy means: we are glad to be together. Someone is glad to be with me!

Right-hemisphere to right-hemisphere communication
- Right brain > left face > left side of retinas > right brain
- Six complete cycles of communication every second
- Synchronized brain chemistry
- Matched brain structure growth
- Authentic, truthful, rapid communication
- Emotions are AMPLIFIED each cycle
- Subjectively experienced as produced by the "other"

Climbing Joy Mountain - Capacity
- Learning to build joy and increase capacity are tasks for the first year of life.

We are created to flow together in rhythms of joy and quiet.

We are creatures of rhythm
- Rhythmic change is our natural state.
- Rhythmic change creates our identity.
- Rhythmic change is the basis for bonding.
- Rhythmic change gives us our strength.

We are created to be deeply connected to each other:
- In times of joy
- In quiet together
- And in the times we feel negative emotions

How do we avoid getting stuck in negative emotions, and learn to return to joy together?

We are created to be together
- Then the Lord God said, "It is not good that man should be alone. I will make him a helper fit for him." Gen 2:18, RSV.
- We are created for each other to help each other!

"Friends always show their love…What are brothers, if not to share trouble?"
- Proverbs. 17:17, Good News Bible.

Spiritual guidelines for building better brains
- Rejoice with those who rejoice
- Weep with those who weep
- Romans 12:15, RSV.

We're one but we're not the same. We get to carry each other.
- From the song "One" by U2 from the "Joshua Tree" CD.

How does our brain learn to return to joy?

Joy means relationship.

Joy means: we are glad to be together. Someone is glad to be with me!

The control center only learns "return to joy" in joyful relationships.
- It needs others to synchronize with it.

CALMING OUR PAINFUL EMOTIONS
RETURNING TO JOY, PART 1: SYNCHRONIZATION & NEGATIVE EMOTIONS

The cingulate cortex is the center for internal and external synchronization
- It is called "The Mother Core."
- The "Mental Banana"
- It is the center for mutual mind.

To learn to return to joy from negative emotions, I need:
- Someone with a well trained banana
  - Who knows how to return to joy from the emotion I feel
- Who is glad to be with me
  - Who has more joy than I have pain and can stay relational with me in spite of my distress
- While I am feeling the negative emotion
  - Who must synchronize with me while I am distressed

Returning to joy and quiet together is a task for the second year of life.
- When I am in distress (I experience one of the Big Six negative emotions.)
- And someone is glad to be with me. (Joy means someone is glad to be with me.)
- And shares my distress (I am able to return to joy since you are glad to be with me.)
- Now we are both feeling distressed but synchronized.
- I can start to quiet myself. (Quiet Together teaches me to quiet myself.)

I learn to self-regulate through mutual regulation
- Both are needed throughout my lifetime
- Mutual regulation is needed for:
  - Learning to return to joy
  - Combining joy strength

The Big Six Negative Emotions
- Anger
- Fear
- Shame
- Disgust
- Sadness
- Hopeless Despair

Pause and discuss: Why did God give us the ability to feel negative emotions?
- Anger
- Fear
- Shame
- Disgust
- Sadness
- Hopeless Despair

EXERCISE: Why Did God Give Us the Ability to Feel Negative Emotions?
25 Minutes

Facilitator Note: Stop the video at this point for the exercise.

The purpose of this exercise is to help participants better understand the purpose for negative emotions by asking the question, "Why did God give us the ability to feel negative emotions?"

CALMING OUR PAINFUL EMOTIONS
RETURNING TO JOY, PART 1: SYNCHRONIZATION & NEGATIVE EMOTIONS

> Recognizing the importance and purpose of negative emotions is very difficult for most people. Many of us have been deeply wounded by others who have acted destructively when feeling negative emotions. We have never seen an example of someone who could handle a negative emotion without someone getting hurt. As a result, negative emotions are a very fearful thing.
>
> The inability to return to joy also makes negative emotions a very painful experience. Getting stuck in a negative emotion hurts, and we can often act out in pain. We can often do or say things that hurt us – or those around us. This may be especially true if we tend to use BEEPS to medicate negative emotions. As a result, we do our best to avoid negative emotions as much as possible.
>
> This exercise is important, because it helps participants recognize that God has created us with the ability to experience negative emotions – for a reason! If we can learn to recognize their purpose, negative emotions can be very constructive. Having a negative emotion can actually be a positive experience, if we can learn to return to joy and respond to it appropriately.

YOUR NOTES

1. Break into small groups of at least 3 people. Your facilitator will help adjust group size depending on the total number of participants.

2. Your facilitator will assign each group one or more of the Big Six Negative Emotions. Each group will spend 10 minutes discussing the reasons why they think God has given them the ability to feel that negative emotion. One member of each group should function as a group secretary, and record everyone's input. Your facilitator will remind you when your discussion time is up.

3. After the small groups have completed their discussions, your facilitator will ask each small group to share the results of their discussions with the entire group. Your facilitator will help moderate this discussion for 10-15 minutes.

4. Following the completion of this exercise, the facilitator will restart the video.

Six basic unpleasant emotions
- Sad: I lost some of my life
- Angry: I need to protect myself and make it stop!
- Frightened: I want to "get away"
- Ashamed: I'm not bringing you joy and/or you are not glad to be with me
- Disgusted: That's not life-giving!
- Hopeless Despair: I lack the time and resources

To self-regulate, my brain must learn to return to joy from every negative emotion
- I must have connections between each negative emotion and joy

Strong connections back to joy from negative emotions must be built
- The connections back to joy from negative emotions must be strong and used frequently.

If the connections back to joy are weak or were never made at all
- For example, suppose that there are no connections back to joy from anger

I'll get stuck in anger when I feel angry
- I won't be able to stay connected to others.

CALMING OUR PAINFUL EMOTIONS
RETURNING TO JOY, PART 1: SYNCHRONIZATION & NEGATIVE EMOTIONS

YOUR NOTES

- I will be consumed with trying to protect myself and make the pain stop.
- I won't act like myself

When we are unsynchronized, we get stuck in negative emotions
- Our level of pain exceeds our level of joy.
- This is experienced as trauma, and results in ongoing emotional distress.
- This is pain at Level 3 of the Control Center.

When we are unsynchronized, joy and relational capacity is low:
- Our level of pain is greater than our level of joy.
- We can't stay connected relationally with others.
- Our relationships tend to break down when we are distressed.
- Our capacity to attach to others in joyful relationships is diminished.

Medicate to regulate

Synchronized relationships increase capacity and the ability to return to joy
- Our level of joy is greater than our level of pain.
- We are able to attach securely to others.
- We have the capacity to stay relational when we are distressed.
- Joyful synchronization creates healthy attachments with God and others.

Next week: Returning To Joy, Part 2
- Synchronization and returning to joy from negative emotions.
- Satan's 2 primary strategies to keep us stuck in pain and relational breakdown.
- Introduction to capacity and attachment.
- Returning to joy, BEEPS and Step 2 of the Twelve Steps.

CLOSE THE GROUP WITH PRAYER

CALMING OUR PAINFUL EMOTIONS
RETURNING TO JOY, PART 1: SYNCHRONIZATION & NEGATIVE EMOTIONS

QUESTIONS FOR FURTHER DISCUSSION OR FOLLOW-UP

1. How did it feel trying to synchronize with others during the walking exercise? How did you feel when others were trying to synchronize with you?

2. Is it hard for you to synchronize with others?

3. Is there anyone in your life that will synchronize with you when you are upset?

4. Why did God create us to be together?

5. How does "Rejoicing with those who rejoice" and Weeping with those who weep" help the brain?

6. What are the three things you need to learn to return to joy from negative emotions?

7. Why is it important that someone else have a well-trained banana if we are going to learn to return to joy? Why is it important that they have a lot of joy strength?

8. How does staying relational help us learn to return to joy from negative emotions?

9. Do you know how to return to joy from the Big Six negative emotions? How long does it take you?

10. What negative emotions do you have the hardest time recovering from?

11. What happens to you when you get stuck in a negative emotion? What happens to your ability to stay connected to others around you?

12. Are you able to act like yourself when you experience the big six negative emotions? If not, how would you like to act when you feel one of these distressing emotions?

13. When you are experiencing one of the Big Six negative emotions, what do you want the most at that time?

14. Do you have a person with a "trained banana" in your life that can help you learn to return to joy from each one of the Big Six negative emotions?

15. Have you ever used BEEPS to medicate one of the Big Six negative emotions? What happened? Did it work?

CALMING OUR PAINFUL EMOTIONS
RETURNING TO JOY, PART 1: SYNCHRONIZATION & NEGATIVE EMOTIONS

OPTIONAL 12 STEP QUESTIONS

1. Many of us who use BEEPS are very uncomfortable with the Big Six negative emotions. Many of us use BEEPS to avoid, minimize or escape these feelings. What do you do when you feel the Big Six negative emotions?
   a. Anger
   b. Fear
   c. Sadness
   d. Shame
   e. Disgust
   f. Hopeless Despair

2. What BEEPS do you use when you feel each of these negative emotions?

3. Do BEEPS help you to return to joy from these negative emotions? What effect do BEEPS have on negative emotions in the long run?

4. Anxiety is the neurochemical equivalent of fear. We are often more aware of feeling anxious than we are of feeling afraid. Do you often feel anxious? What does your body feel like when you are anxious?

5. What happens to you when your anxiety builds? What do you feel?

6. What happens to your relationships when your anxiety grows?

7. What BEEPS do you use to relieve growing feelings of anxiety?

8. Do BEEPS make you feel less anxious?

9. What have you found that works to help you feel less anxious?

10. Have you found anything that helps you when you are experiencing a Big Six negative emotion?

11. Are you able to effectively handle negative emotions by yourself?

12. How did people in your house handle the Big Six negative emotions when you were growing up?

13. How do you feel when others around you are experiencing one of the Big Six distressing negative emotions?

14. Do you feel powerless over negative emotions?

15. Does just thinking and talking about negative emotions raise your level of anxiety?

16. Do you like how you act when you feel distressing emotions – or do you find yourself doing and saying things that you feel ashamed of later?

17. Do negative emotions make your life unmanageable?

18. What does the expression "emotionally sober" mean to you? Is it possible to be sober from the use of BEEPS – and still not be emotionally sober? Why or why not?

4 STRATEGIES THAT KEEP YOU STUCK
RETURNING TO JOY, PART 2: CAPACITY, ATTACHMENT & BEEPS

OPEN THE GROUP

- Ask for a volunteer to open the group in prayer.

EXERCISE: THE BIG SIX EMOTIONS. *15 Minutes*

Facilitator Note: This exercise is designed to help participants review the Big Six negative emotions from last week's lesson. It will also help participants begin to think about how they can apply Restarting materials to their daily experience.

The facilitator can best help participants review these definitions by demonstrating what each negative emotion looks like. For example, when defining the negative emotion of shame (I'm not bringing you joy and/or you are not glad to be with me), you can illustrate this emotion by looking at the floor, letting your shoulders sag, and covering your face with your hands. Acting out each negative emotion as you review the definitions gives the participants a right-brain illustration of the concepts you are helping them learn. Be creative and have fun with this! Make sure that you do not overwhelm participants by acting out extremely intense examples of these emotions.

1. Break into small groups of 3 people.

2. Your facilitator will remind you of the definitions of the Big Six negative emotions from last week's lesson. These emotions are:
   a. Sad: I lost some of my life.
   b. Angry: I need to protect myself and make it stop!
   c. Frightened: I want to "get away."
   d. Ashamed: I'm not bringing you joy and/or you are not glad to be with me.
   e. Disgusted: That's not life-giving!
   f. Hopeless Despair: I lack the time and resources.

3. Each person in the small groups will have 3 minutes to share what they learned about synchronization and the Big Six negative emotions from last week's lesson. If what you learned made a positive difference in how you handled a negative emotion in the past week, you are encouraged to share your experience.

4. Remember to stay relational as you share:
   a. Maintain appropriate eye contact.
   b. Support each other through active listening.
   c. Please do not offer criticism or advice after others have shared.

5. Your facilitator will keep track of time for you so that everyone in your group has a chance to share.

6. When this exercise is complete, your facilitator will remind you to gather into a large group for this week's lesson.

STRATEGIES THAT KEEP YOU STUCK
RETURNING TO JOY, PART 2: CAPACITY, ATTACHMENT & BEEPS

YOUR NOTES

TODAY'S LESSON: Returning to Joy, Part 2
Capacity, Attachment and BEEPS

> **Facilitator Note:** Play Session Four on the Restarting DVD.
> - Ask the class to follow along in their workbooks, and take notes as needed.
> - The final segment of this video contains instructions on how to tell Level 4+ Joy Stories. In the final exercise of this session, participants will have the opportunity to practice telling Level 4+ Joy Stories.

CLASS NOTES: Returning to Joy, Part 2.
Capacity, Attachment and BEEPS

A quick review:

Learning to flow together in rhythms of joy and quiet is a task for the first year of life.

Returning to joy and quiet together is a task for the second year of life.
- When I am in distress (I experience one of the Big Six negative emotions).
- And someone is glad to be with me (Joy means someone is glad to be with me).
- And shares my distress (I am able to Return to Joy since you are glad to be with me).
- Now we are both feeling distressed but synchronized
- I can start to quiet myself (Quiet Together teaches me to quiet myself).

The control center only learns "Return to Joy" in joyful relationships
- It needs others to synchronize with it.

To learn to return to joy from negative emotions, I need:
- Someone with a well trained banana.
  - Who knows how return to joy from the emotion I feel.
- Who is glad to be with me
  - Who has more joy than I have pain and can stay relational with me in spite of my distress.
- While I am feeling the negative emotion.
  - Must synchronize with me while I am distressed.

The Big Six negative emotions
- Anger
- Fear
- Shame
- Disgust
- Sadness
- Hopeless Despair

To self-regulate, my brain must learn to return to joy from every negative emotion.
- I must have connections between each negative emotion and joy.

Strong connections back to joy from negative emotions must be built.
- The connections back to joy from negative emotions must be strong and used frequently.

STRATEGIES THAT KEEP YOU STUCK
RETURNING TO JOY, PART 2: CAPACITY, ATTACHMENT & BEEPS

If the connections back to joy are weak or were never made at all...
- For example, suppose that there are no connections back to joy from anger.

I'll get stuck in anger when I feel angry:
- I won't be able to stay connected to others.
- I will be consumed with trying to protect myself and make the pain stop.
- I won't act like myself.

When we are unsynchronized, we get stuck in negative emotions:
- Our level of pain exceeds our level of joy.
- This is experienced as trauma, and results in ongoing emotional distress.
- This is pain at Level 3 of the Control Center.

Synchronized relationships increase capacity and the ability to return to joy:
- Our level of joy is greater than our level of pain.
- We are able to attach securely to others.
- We have the capacity to stay relational when we are distressed.
- Joyful synchronization creates healthy attachments with God and others.

When we are unsynchronized, joy and relational capacity is low:
- Our level of pain is greater than our level of joy.
- We can't stay connected relationally with others.
- Our relationships tend to break down when we are distressed.
- Our capacity to attach to others in joyful relationships is diminished.

Satan has 2 primary strategies to keep us stuck in pain and relational breakdown:
- To cause us to live our lives from pain.
- To live our lives from "The Sark."

There is one strategy for each hemisphere of the brain
- The right hemisphere
  - Pain: the pusher
- The left hemisphere
  - Sark: the picker

Pain: the pusher
- Pain in the control center means that life and relationships will be pain-driven (pushed by pain).
- Eliminating, avoiding or medicating pain becomes our most important need and motivation.
- Relationship with God is mostly about trying to eliminate, hide, avoid or medicate pain.
- Relationships with others are about avoiding, hiding or using others to relieve or medicate pain.

The sark: the picker
- The mistaken belief that we are able to pick the right and wrong course of action for our lives – one that will not hurt.
- Explanations for life, good and evil are based on the drive to eliminate, medicate or avoid pain.
- We are consumed with knowing good and evil – not God.
- It is stubborn, persistent and always wrong!

YOUR NOTES

STRATEGIES THAT KEEP YOU STUCK
RETURNING TO JOY, PART 2: CAPACITY, ATTACHMENT & BEEPS

The sark is driven by the mistaken belief that it can pick the right or wrong thing to do.
- The Sark is absolutely opposed to the Spirit of God. Romans 8: 6-9.

The biblically informed sark is especially problematic
- It is what crucified Jesus.

Pain and sark driven belief systems guide our understanding of good and evil.
- If it hurts, it is bad and must not be God.
- If it is less painful, it is good and must be God.
- If I serve God and it is painful:
  - It can't be God's will.
  - I must be wrong.
  - God and/or others don't care about me.
- If I serve God and it is not painful:
  - It must be God's will.
  - I must be right.
  - God and others do care.

Through pain and the sark, our capacity for joy is diminished
- Our level of pain exceeds our level of joy.
- We live in pain, feel separated from God and others and can't stay relational with them.
- These are the goals of Satan's strategies.
- We cannot securely attach to God and others in joyful relationships.

Synchronization creates capacity and attachment.

There are four types of attachments:
- Secure
- Dismissive
- Distracted
- Disorganized

BEEPS
- BEEPS are attachments to Behaviors, Events, Experiences, People or Substances that are used to regulate emotions, increase pleasure or decrease pain.

BEEPS
- Attachments to BEEPS help us medicate – to artificially regulate – positive and negative emotions as well as pain.

BEEPS
- Attachments to BEEPS take the place of secure attachments to God and significant others.

BEEPS
- There are many different types of BEEPS. Examples can include:
- Behaviors: Work
- Events: Thrill Seeking
- Experiences: Sex
- People: Relationships
- Substances: Alcohol

STRATEGIES THAT KEEP YOU STUCK
RETURNING TO JOY, PART 2: CAPACITY, ATTACHMENT & BEEPS

YOUR NOTES

The Twelve Steps and return to joy
- Step 2: Came to believe that a power greater than ourselves could restore us to sanity.

BEEPS and Return to Joy:
- When we use BEEPS to avoid or regulate negative emotions, our negative emotions become wired to BEEPS.
- This means that negative emotions will powerfully trigger the drive to use BEEPS.
- It becomes almost impossible to avoid BEEPS when triggered.

This wiring between negative emotions and BEEPS are part of the insanity of BEEPS:
- We do the same things, over and over again, and expect different results.
- But because our wiring doesn't change, we are triggered by the same feelings and get the same result: BEEPS!

When we feel a negative emotion like hopeless despair:
- We use BEEPS to medicate it, until we don't feel distressed, or the level of pleasure from BEEPS covers our level of pain.

We need a power greater than ourselves who can restore us to sanity…
- We need God – and others:
  - With well trained brains
  - Who are empowered by joy
  - Who know how to handle the emotion
  - Who are glad to be with us in our distress

That's how we learn to return to joy and stay relational with each other!

LEARNING TO TELL LEVEL 4+ JOY STORIES

> **Facilitator Note:** The material that follows introduces Level 4+ Joy Stories, and teaches participants how to tell Level 4+ Joy Stories. Participants will practice telling these joyful stories.

These materials are from:
- "The Life Model: Living from the Heart Jesus Gave You." By Dr. E. James Wilder and others.
- Level 4+ slides are from "THRIVE Sensible Strategies" by Chris and Jen Coursey, © 2006.

Level 4+ Stories:
- Include both the left and right hemispheres of the brain
- Provide examples of how we are to act when upset
- Give us practice – the more we tell, the better we become
- Help us use words for emotions and body sensations
- Give us opportunity to gather emotion stories for use at other times with other people
- Give us opportunity to critique others' stories and receive feedback. This improves mind sight
- Build our capacity to return to joy from distress and increase our ability to regulate our own emotions
- Illustrate how others act like themselves

STRATEGIES THAT KEEP YOU STUCK
RETURNING TO JOY, PART 2: CAPACITY, ATTACHMENT & BEEPS

- Spark memories to find our own stories
- Build bonds and create a group identity

Characteristics of Level 4+ stories
- Describe what your body feels during the emotions
- It must be a story you have told before
- Use enough words to describe what is occurring from your point of view
  Let the listeners into "your world" descriptively
- Use feeling words to describe body sensations
- Make it autobiographical; you are involved
- State specifically how you like to act during the emotion
- Maintain eye contact (stay relational) during the story telling

Level 4+ story Guidelines
- Pick a story you do not need to be guarded in telling
- The story must illustrate and evoke the feeling
- Show the authentic emotion in your voice and face
- Do not pick an intense story – rather, find one with a medium feeling level

4+ Synchronized story Summary
- Use enough words for others to understand easily
- Use feeling words for sensations and emotions
- Be autobiographical; you are involved
- Maintain eye contact during story telling
- Stay relational
- Show authentic emotions on your face and in your voice
- Describe how your body feels during the emotions
- Tell specifically how you like to act during the emotions

Preparing My Level 4+ Story Worksheet
1. This story has a moderate feeling level and is not too intense
2. I have told this story before
3. I do not need to be guarded in telling this story
4. This story is autobiographical (I am involved in the story)
5. This story illustrates a specific feeling
6. I will show the authentic emotion on my face and in my voice
7. I will maintain eye contact while storytelling
8. Briefly describe the situation:
9. Feeling words for this story:
10. During this story my body felt:
11. The things I did in this story that demonstrate how I like to act in this emotion are (or if I did not act like myself at the time, it would have been like me to do this…)

Follow your level 4+ story worksheet as you listen Ed's Level 4+ Joy Story.

Tell a Level 4+ Joy Story!

STRATEGIES THAT KEEP YOU STUCK
RETURNING TO JOY, PART 2: CAPACITY, ATTACHMENT & BEEPS

EXERCISE: LEARNING TO TELL A LEVEL 4+ JOY STORY *30 Minutes*

Facilitator Notes: Level 4+ stories are a powerful way to build capacity and joy. As you will discover in the coming weeks, Level 4+ stories are used to describe a variety of experiences and emotions. In this exercise, participant will have the opportunity to learn and practice telling a Level 4+ story about a joyful experience. An introduction to Level 4+ stories and an example of a Level 4+ story are provided on this week's video.

These stories are called Level 4+ stories because they involve all 4 levels of the emotional control center in the right hemisphere of the brain – plus the verbal left hemisphere. In these stories, participants describe a specific experience, and the emotions and body sensations they felt during the experience. Using words to tell the story involves the left hemisphere of the brain. Describing the emotions and body sensations involves the right hemisphere of the brain, which is dominant for emotions and body sensations.

To complete this exercise, participants will need to locate the "Preparing My Level 4+ Joy Story" worksheet in their workbook.

To help participants learn to tell Level 4+ stories, it is helpful to do several things. First, review the worksheet so that participants understand how to complete it. As you review the worksheet, you can use Ed's Level 4+ Joy Story to help participants recognize the elements of a Level 4+ story. Second, tell your own Level 4+ story! The best way for participants to learn to tell Level 4+ stories is for them to hear one. Finally, after you tell your story, ask participants to give you feedback to help you discover how well your story met the guidelines for a Level 4+ story listed on the worksheet.

You can help your group learn to give Level 4+ story feedback by reviewing your story and the guidelines with them. To do this, start with the first characteristic listed on the worksheet, and ask the group if your story was moderate in feeling – or too intense. Listen to their feedback. Continue this process until you have reviewed and received feedback for each Level 4+ story characteristic. Modeling this process is important for participants, because it teaches them how to give and receive Level 4+ story feedback. It also helps them better understand the characteristics of a Level 4+ story.

When you have completed your story and received feedback, it is time for participants to complete their own Level 4+ story worksheet. After you have given them 5 minutes to complete the worksheets, volunteers may begin sharing their stories in small group. Volunteers will have 3 minutes to share their story, followed by 2 minutes of feedback. Be sure to keep track of time so that each person has enough time to share and receive feedback.

Before the groups begin sharing, it is a good idea to ask participants to raise their hands if they get stuck, have questions or need help once small group sharing begins. Be ready to help as needed.

1. Break into small groups of 3 people.

2. Take 5 minutes to complete the "Preparing My 4+ Story Worksheet" that is in your workbook. Your facilitator will review the worksheet with you and may use Ed's Level 4+ Joy Story from the video to help you recognize the elements and characteristics of a Level 4+ story.

STRATEGIES THAT KEEP YOU STUCK
RETURNING TO JOY, PART 2: CAPACITY, ATTACHMENT & BEEPS

a. Please make sure that your story is not so emotionally intense that it overwhelms others.
b. It helps if this is a story that you have told before – this makes it easier to share.
c. It is a good idea to avoid stories that may cause you or others feelings of shame or embarrassment.
d. Make sure that the story is about your feelings and that you are involved in the story.
e. Be sure that your story clearly illustrates a specific feeling.
f. As you tell your story, let your face and voice reflect the emotion you are describing.
g. As you maintain eye contact with others in your small group, it will help you stay connected relationally with them.
h. Write a brief description of the situation you want to share. You only need to write down enough details to help you remember the story – and be able to share it.
i. Write the feeling words that describe the emotions that you felt during the story. It helps to list each one.
j. Write down how your body felt during the situation you are describing. It may be things like: "my stomach was in a knot" or "my shoulders felt tight" or "my muscles felt relaxed."
k. Describe what you did in the situation that illustrates how you like to act when you are feeling that specific emotion. What is it like you to do when you are feeling great joy? Maybe you like to tell others how excited you feel – or perhaps you like to say a quick "thanks" to God. If you didn't act like yourself when you had the feeling you are describing, what would it have been like you to do?

3. Your facilitator will tell a Level 4+ Joy Story.

4. Your facilitator will ask you for feedback that describes how well their Level 4+ story met the guidelines listed on your worksheet.
   a. Locate the guidelines for Level 4+ stories on your worksheet.
   b. Your facilitator will read the first characteristic of a Level 4+ story.
   c. Your facilitator will ask you if the story met that guideline, and listen to your feedback.
   d. Your facilitator will repeat this process until they have received feedback based on every Level 4+ story characteristic.

5. Take 5 minutes and complete the worksheet for your own Level 4+ story. Your facilitator will help you by keeping track of time.

6. Your facilitator will ask for volunteers in each small group to begin telling a Level 4+ Joy Story. You will have 3 minutes to tell your story. Your facilitator will keep track of time for you. If at any point your group gets stuck or has a question, please raise your hand, and your facilitator will come help you.

7. After the first joy story, each group can take 2 minutes to give feedback on the story. Use the "Preparing My 4+ Story Worksheet" as a guideline to help the story teller discover if they were able to share all the elements of a 4+ story that are listed on the worksheet. Be encouraging and positive! Your facilitator will keep track of time for you, and let you know when it is time for the next person to share their story.

8. Your facilitator will let you know when it is time for a second person in each small group to begin their 3-minute Level 4+ Joy Story, followed by 2 minutes of feedback.

STRATEGIES THAT KEEP YOU STUCK
RETURNING TO JOY, PART 2: CAPACITY, ATTACHMENT & BEEPS

YOUR NOTES

Your facilitator will keep track of time for you and let you know when it is time for the next person to share their story.

9. Your facilitator will let you know when it is time for the third person in each small group to begin their 3-minute Level 4+ Joy Story, followed by 2 minutes of feedback. Your facilitator will keep track of time for you.

10. At the conclusion of the exercise, your facilitator may ask volunteers to share about their experience with the entire group. Use one word to describe how it felt to share and hear joy stories.

CLOSE THE GROUP WITH PRAYER

STRATEGIES THAT KEEP YOU STUCK
RETURNING TO JOY, PART 2: CAPACITY, ATTACHMENT & BEEPS

QUESTIONS FOR FURTHER DISCUSSION OR FOLLOW-UP

1. Have you noticed a difference in how you think about or deal with negative emotions in the past week? What if anything is different?

2. Can you imagine what it would be like to stay connected to others when you experience a negative emotion? How would you act? What would it feel like?

3. What are Satan's two primary strategies to keep us stuck in pain and relational breakdown?

4. When you are stuck in pain, what do you spend most of your time trying to do? How does this affect you – and your relationships?

5. Is your relationship with God different when you are feeling a lot of pain? How does it change?

6. What does living in pain "push" you to do?

7. How do you define "The Sark?"

8. What is it about your own sark that keeps you stuck? How does your sark affect you?

9. Are you able to pick the right thing or wrong thing to do in your life? Why?

10. Why is it so hard to realize that our sark is always wrong?

11. What belief systems in your life are pain and sark driven? How do these keep you stuck?

12. What are the four attachment styles? Briefly describe each one.

13. What does Step 2 mean to you? Describe it in your own words.

14. Why do we need to be restored to sanity when we use BEEPS to regulate negative emotions?

15. Has the statement been true in your life? "We use BEEPS to medicate until we don't feel distressed or the level of pleasure from BEEPS covers our level of pain." Explain.

16. What do we need to be restored to sanity?

17. Can you break the strength of BEEPS attachments by sheer willpower? Why or why not?

18. Do you think that learning to tell Level 4+ Joy Stories can help increase your joy capacity? Explain.

STRATEGIES THAT KEEP YOU STUCK
RETURNING TO JOY, PART 2: CAPACITY, ATTACHMENT & BEEPS

OPTIONAL 12 STEP QUESTIONS

1. What is Step 2? Describe it in your own words.

2. Insanity has been described as "Doing the same thing, over and over again, and expecting a different result." Has this been true of your relationship with BEEPS?

3. Can you remember a time when you decided that you wanted to stop using a BEEPS – and really meant it – only to find that you used BEEPS again anyway? Describe this event.
   a. What BEEPS were you using?
   b. Why did you decide to stop using? What happened to cause you to make this decision?
   c. What actions did you take to stop using?
   d. What happened just before you used again?
   e. What emotions were you feeling just before you used again?
   f. What was your body feeling just before you used again?
   g. What happened when you used BEEPS again?
   h. What emotions did you feel afterwards – and in the next few days?
   i. How many times did you repeat this cycle?

4. Have you ever used more than one BEEPS to help medicate your feelings?

5. Have you ever stopped using one BEEPS, and then started or increased the use of another? Did this solve anything?

6. What has happened to relationships that are important to you when you tried to stop using BEEPS, and relapsed back into them? List each relationship that was affected.

7. What happens to your feelings about yourself when you try to stop using BEEPS – and can't?

8. Have you ever asked God to help you stop BEEPS? What happened?

9. Did you ever feel angry or disappointed with God after you asked Him for help – and then used again later?

10. Are you capable of changing the wiring between BEEPS and negative emotions in your brain?

11. Do you have specific negative emotions that are wired to BEEPS? What are they?

12. Have you ever tried to avoid specific negative emotions so that you would not use BEEPS? Have you been able to successfully avoid them? List each emotion you've tried to avoid – and your strategy for avoiding each.

13. Has your willpower alone been enough to change your attachments with BEEPS? Why?

14. What do you need to be restored back to sanity? Be specific.

15. Where can you go to find this help?

PREPARING MY 4+ JOY STORY WORKSHEET

1. This story has a moderate feeling level and is not too intense ☐

2. I have told this story before ☐

3. I do not need to be guarded in telling this story ☐

4. This story is autobiographical (I am involved in the story) ☐

5. This story illustrates a specific feeling ☐

6. I will show the authentic emotion on my face and in my voice ☐

7. I will maintain eye contact while storytelling ☐

8. Briefly describe the situation:

9. Feeling words for this story:

10. During this story my body felt:

11. The things I did in this story that demonstrate how I like to act in this emotion are (or if I did not act like myself at the time, it would have been like me to do this…)

5 HEALTHY RELATIONSHIPS
WHAT IS SECURE ATTACHMENT?

OPEN THE GROUP

- Ask for a volunteer to open the group in prayer.

EXERCISE: A LEVEL 4+ JOY STORY *15 Minutes*

Facilitator Note: As we learned last week, Level 4+ stories are a powerful way to build capacity and joy. In this exercise, two volunteers will have the opportunity to practice telling a Level 4+ Joy Story to the entire group. For the sake of time, it is easier if volunteers tell the Level 4+ story they shared with their group last week.

These stories are called Level 4+ stories because they involve all 4 levels of the emotional control center in the right hemisphere of the brain – plus the verbal left hemisphere. In these stories, participants describe a specific experience, and the emotions and body sensations they felt during the experience. Using words to tell the story involves the left hemisphere of the brain. Describing the emotions and body sensations involves the right hemisphere of the brain, which is dominant for emotions and body sensations.

Before volunteers begin their stories, it is helpful to use the guidelines for Level 4+ stories from last week's worksheet to review the characteristics of Level 4+ stories. Since volunteers are sharing stories from last week's lesson, it is not necessary to give detailed instructions about how to complete the worksheet or tell Level 4+ stories.

Be very encouraging and supportive as you ask two volunteers to share their stories. As with last week's exercise, volunteers will have 3 minutes to tell their story. After they have completed their story, it is important that you moderate 2 minutes of feedback from the group about the story. As with feedback in last week's exercise, go through each element of a 4+ story as listed on the worksheet one at a time, and ask participants if the volunteer's story contained each element. Please remind everyone that feedback on Level 4+ stories focuses on making sure the story contained all the elements of a 4+ story as described on the worksheet.

It is very important that you affirm and encourage each volunteer who shares with the entire group.

1. The facilitator will ask two volunteers to share a Level 4+ Joy Story with the entire group.

2. Due to time constraints, volunteers are encouraged to share their joy story from last week.

3. Be sure to stay relational while telling the story.

4. Each story should be limited to 3 minutes. Your facilitator will help you keep track of time.

HEALTHY RELATIONSHIPS
WHAT IS SECURE ATTACHMENT ?

YOUR NOTES

5. After each story, the facilitator and group will have the opportunity to give feedback. Use the "Preparing My 4+ Story Worksheet" as a guideline to help the storyteller discover if he/she was able to share all the elements of a 4+ story listed on the worksheet. Be encouraging and positive! Feedback should last for 2 minutes, and your facilitator will keep track of time for you.

TODAY'S LESSON: What is a Secure Attachment?

Facilitator Note: Play Session Five on the Restarting DVD.
- Ask the class to follow along in their workbooks, and take notes as needed.
- Please note that you will need to stop the video several times to lead exercises. The video will let you know when to stop.

CLASS NOTES: What is a Secure Attachment?

When attachment is secure, life is powered by joy.
- We can synchronize with each other.
- We can bond and work together in joy.
- We fulfill our purpose and destiny together!

God created us to securely attach to Him and each other in joy!

We are created for relationship with God.
- Then God said, "Let Us make man in Our image, according to Our likeness… So God created man in His own image; in the image of God He created him; male and female He created them. Then God saw everything that He had made, and indeed it was very good. Genesis 1:26, 27, 31. NKJV
- God worked with Adam to name animals. Genesis 2:7.
- God walked with Adam and Eve in the cool part of the day. Genesis 3:8.

Even if we're stuck in negative emotions, or don't feel good enough to attach to Him, or struggle with things we feel ashamed of, God is totally committed to joyful relationship with us.

Jesus said:
- "Behold, I stand at the door and knock. If anyone hears My voice and opens the door, I will come in to him and dine with him, and he with Me."

Revelation 3:20 NKJV.

We are also created for secure attachment to each other.
- …And the Lord God said, "It is not good that man should be alone; I will make him a helper comparable to him…He brought her to the man. And Adam said: "This is now bone of my bones and flesh of my flesh…Therefore a man shall leave his father and mother and be joined to his wife, and they shall become one flesh." And they were both naked, the man and his wife, and were not ashamed.

Genesis 2:18, 23-25, NKJV.

HEALTHY RELATIONSHIPS
WHAT IS SECURE ATTACHMENT ?

Secure attachment means:
- Adam and Eve experienced joyful relationship with God and each other.
- They were synchronized together in rhythms of joy and quiet together.
- Securely bonded intimately for life.
- They could fulfill their purpose and destiny together.

Why do we need secure attachment to be fulfilled?
- What did God create us to do?

Be fruitful and multiply
- Bring and give life wherever you go.

Subdue, have dominion, rule
- Take relationships and Eden to places they've never been.

Serve, steward and work
- Maintain and guard what we've been given.

Protect, serve and enjoy family as mature parents
- Pass on to the next generation what I've been given.

Experience and enjoy pleasure together
- The word "Eden" means "Pleasure."

Learn truth in joyful relationships
- Know God and each other – not good and evil.

Choose who we will serve
- God, each other – or ourselves.

We are created with each of these desires, drives and purposes
- And we are designed to be completely fulfilled only in joyful, secure relationships with God and each other.

What happens when we are not securely attached?
- What is attachment pain?

Attachment pain is distress at level 1 of the emotional control center in the right hemisphere of the brain.
- It is the deepest level of pain.

Level 1 attachment pain:
- Attachment pain is the deepest level of pain.
- It is sub-cortical – below our conscious awareness.
- It results from insecure or disorganized attachments.
- It is what we feel when we don't know where we belong or have someone to belong to.
- It is what we feel when we don't know who and what is personal to me.
- It pervades and affects every area of life.
- Everything hurts!

YOUR NOTES

HEALTHY RELATIONSHIPS
WHAT IS SECURE ATTACHMENT ?

YOUR NOTES

EXERCISE: ATTACHMENT PAIN AND POPULAR MUSIC *5 Minutes*

Facilitator Note: Please stop the video at this point for the exercise.

As mentioned in the facilitator's notes at the beginning of this chapter, attachment pain is sub-cortical, and below our level of conscious awareness. This can make it very difficult to recognize.

This exercise asks facilitator and participants to share song titles – or words – that have a theme of attachment pain. This is a fun and relatively non-threatening way to learn to identify attachment pain – and what it feels like. To prepare for this exercise, you should spend some time thinking about songs that contain an attachment pain theme. It is helpful to share a few of these songs at the beginning of the exercise. After sharing your favorite attachment pain songs or lyrics, encourage participants to share any attachment pain songs they know.

Singing is not required – but may be optional – if participants are adventurous. Have fun with this exercise!

1. Because attachment pain is sub-cortical, it is below our level of conscious awareness, and is often very difficult to recognize. This exercise is a fun way to learn to identify and describe attachment pain – and what it feels like.
2. Your facilitator will begin by sharing a few of his/her favorite songs with a theme of attachment pain with the entire group.
3. Volunteers can then take turns sharing their favorite attachment pain songs and lyrics with the entire group. This can be a lot of fun – and singing is not required! What songs about attachment pain do you know, and what stories do they tell?
4. Your facilitator will help you keep track of time, and will turn the DVD back on when the exercise is complete.

Facilitator Note: Restart the video.

Attachment pain
- If joy is shared, attachment grows even when you planned and agreed not to do so.
- Makes good solutions turn sour or sexual.
- Adds intensity to everything at higher levels and should be suspected when solutions to obvious higher level problems do not work.
- Drives cutting and other addictions like food.

EXERCISE: HOW BADLY DOES ATTACHMENT PAIN HURT? *5 Minutes*

Facilitator Note: Please stop the video at this point for the exercise.

Because attachment pain tends to be unrecognized, many of us have never developed a vocabulary to describe how bad it feels. This exercise helps participants learn to use feeling words to describe the distress of attachment pain. It is helpful if you begin this exercise by sharing a few feeling words that describe how attachment pain feels to you.

HEALTHY RELATIONSHIPS
WHAT IS SECURE ATTACHMENT ?

> You may also use feelings expressed in songs from the first exercise to describe attachment pain.
>
> In this exercise, it is important to share only one or two word descriptions of attachment pain. Limiting descriptions to one or two words helps keep the group from being overwhelmed by detailed and graphic illustrations of the distress associated with attachment pain.
>
> After you have shared a few examples with the group, ask volunteers from the group to share their own one or two word descriptions of attachment pain. They can share either what attachment pain feels like to them – or feelings expressed in songs from the first exercise.
>
> Be sensitive to the pain level of your group. If you feel that the pain level is getting too high, you may shorten the length of this exercise.

1. Because attachment pain is below our conscious level of awareness, it is often very difficult to describe what it feels like. Sometimes, we don't even have words to describe that level of pain. This exercise can help us learn new feeling words that can help us describe and better understand attachment pain.
2. Your as the facilitator will start by giving a few one or two word examples that describe how attachment pain feels. Your facilitator may share:
   a. His/her own feelings of attachment pain
   b. Feelings of attachment pain described in the songs from the previous exercise
3. Your facilitator will ask volunteers to share one or two word descriptions that illustrate the feeling of attachment pain. Please limit your responses to one or two words only. This will help everyone from being overwhelmed by overly intense descriptions of attachment pain.
4. Your facilitator will help you keep track of time, and will turn the DVD back on when the exercise is complete.

Facilitator Note: Restart the video.

Unrecognized attachment pain
- Recognition and interpretation are learned
- Addictions and the nucleus accumbens
- Masturbation
- Quick fixes and "miracle" breakthroughs are seen as the way out. Long-term healing relationships with God and others are seen as unnecessary, unimportant or "unspiritual."
- Rescuing and over-involvement
- Mistaken attempts at "therapeutic parenting" because attachment pain – not the needs of the child – drive it.

YOUR NOTES

HEALTHY RELATIONSHIPS
WHAT IS SECURE ATTACHMENT ?

YOUR NOTES

EXERCISE: CAN ATTACHMENT PAIN LEAD TO BEEPS? *5 Minutes*

Facilitator Note: Please stop the video at this point for the exercise.

Attachment pain frequently is the unrecognized pain that drives attachments to BEEPS. This exercise is designed to help participants understand the connections between attachment pain and BEEPS. You do not need to tell a Level 4+ story in this exercise.

To begin the exercise, you will need to share examples of the BEEPS – attachment pain connection with participants. You can do this in one of two ways.

First, you can share about a moment in your life when you used BEEPS to medicate attachment pain. To do this, share what the attachment pain felt like in a few words and then describe what BEEPS you used. It is not necessary to go into a detailed description of the attachment pain, or your experience with BEEPS. Simply helping participants realize that there is a connection between attachment pain and BEEPS is enough.

A second way you can illustrate the connection between attachment pain and BEEPS is through popular music. Popular music is filled with references to attachment pain – and the Behaviors, Events, Experiences, People and Substances that are used to medicate it. If you choose this option, prepare in advance by thinking about or searching for songs that illustrate this connection. You may share the song or lyrics with your group.

After you have shared examples of the relationship between attachment pain and BEEPS, volunteers may begin sharing any songs they know that illustrate the connections between attachment pain and BEEPS. You may also ask volunteers to raise their hands if they have ever used BEEPS to relieve attachment pain. It is not necessary to ask volunteers to share the details of their attachment pain or usage of BEEPS in this exercise.

1. Attachment pain frequently is the unrecognized pain that drives attachments to BEEPS. This exercise can help you recognize the connections between attachment pain and BEEPS. You do not need to tell a Level 4+ story in this exercise.
2. Your facilitator will give you a few examples of the connection between attachment pain and BEEPS. Your facilitator may:
   a. Share about a time in which he/she felt attachment pain and used BEEPS to medicate it. He/she will use a few words to describe their attachment pain, and then what BEEPS he/she used.
   b. Share a few examples of songs that illustrate the connection between attachment pain and BEEPS.
3. Your facilitator will ask volunteers to share any songs they know that illustrate the connections between attachment pain and BEEPS.
4. Your facilitator may ask if anyone in the group has ever used BEEPS to medicate attachment pain.
   a. You may respond to this question only if you feel comfortable doing so.
   b. Volunteers may answer "yes" by raising their hands.
5. Your facilitator will help you keep track of time, and will turn the DVD back on when the exercise is complete.

Facilitator Note: Restart the video.

HEALTHY RELATIONSHIPS
WHAT IS SECURE ATTACHMENT ?

We are created to attach to God and others.
- If attachment is broken – or not secure, we will attach to someone or something to make the pain stop.

Medicate to regulate

BEEPS
- BEEPS are attachments to Behaviors, Events, Experiences, People or Substances that are used to regulate emotions, increase pleasure or decrease pain.

BEEPS
- Attachments to BEEPS help us medicate – to artificially regulate – positive and negative emotions as well as pain.

BEEPS
- Attachments to BEEPS take the place of secure attachments to God and significant others.

BEEPS
- There are many different types of BEEPS. Examples can include:
- Behaviors: Work
- Events: Thrill Seeking
- Experiences: Sex
- People: Relationships
- Substances: Alcohol

BEEPS and attachment pain bring us:
- Absolute powerlessness
  - We are incapable of fixing the problem. It is simply too big.
- Absolute unmanageability
  - No matter how hard we try, our lives are totally out of control.
- Absolute insanity
  - Our emotions and logic are hopelessly distorted. We live in pain – but deny the reality of the problem – and blame everyone but BEEPS!

Secure attachment and the Twelve Steps
- Step 3: Made a decision to turn our will and our lives over to the care of God as we understood Him.

When I turn my will and life over to the care of Jesus:
- He attaches to me in absolute and complete joy.
- My life will not be the same!

YOUR NOTES

HEALTHY RELATIONSHIPS
WHAT IS SECURE ATTACHMENT ?

EXERCISE: TELL A LEVEL 4+ STORY ABOUT SECURE ATTACHMENT
35 Minutes

Facilitator Note: In last week's lesson, participants learned to tell Level 4+ stories by describing an experience that was joyful. In this exercise, participants will focus on telling a Level 4+ story about an experience with secure attachment.

As we learned last week, Level 4+ stories are a great way to help build joyful capacity and bonds. Level 4+ stories involve all four levels of the emotional control center in the right hemisphere of the brain – plus the verbal left hemisphere. You may find it helpful to review the facilitator notes and instructions for Level 4+ stories in last week's lesson prior to leading this exercise. It is also a good idea to go over the characteristics of a Level 4+ story listed on your "Preparing My Level 4+ Secure Attachment Story" worksheet, which is located in your workbook.

Start this exercise by sharing a few words that describe how secure attachments with God and others feel to you. Volunteers may then share one-word descriptions of how secure attachments feel to them. Beginning the exercise like this helps participants begin to reflect on experiences they may have had with secure attachment that can be used in their Level 4+ stories.

To help participants prepare to tell their Level 4+ Secure Attachment Story, it is helpful to do several things. First, make sure participants locate their "Preparing My Level 4+ Secure Attachment Story" worksheet in their workbook. Briefly review each characteristic of a Level 4+ story listed on the worksheet with them.

Second, tell your own Level 4+ story about secure attachment. The best way for participants to learn to tell a Level 4+ Secure Attachment Story is to hear one. It is important that you tell this story based on an actual experience that you had with a securely attached person. It is likely that some participants have never had a relationship with a securely attached person. For this reason, it is very important that you describe your emotions, body sensations and behavior in your secure attachment experience.

Please be aware that participants who have never had an experience with a securely attached person will have several options as they tell their 4+ story. First, they may describe a time in their relationship with God in which they experienced secure attachment. Second, if they have never experienced secure attachment in their relationship with God or another person, they may tell a story describing how they think they would feel and act in a securely attached relationship.

Third, ask your group to help you determine if your story met all the guidelines for Level 4+ stories listed on the worksheet. Read each characteristic listed on the worksheet, and then ask your group if your Level 4+ story met each one. It is helpful to remind your group that feedback on Level 4+ stories does not include comments, criticisms or advice based on an experience or feelings shared during a story. Feedback is based solely on the worksheet guidelines.

When feedback is complete, it is time for participants to take 5 minutes and complete their own Level 4+ Secure Attachment Story worksheet. When they are finished, volunteers may begin sharing their stories with their small group. Volunteers will have 3 minutes to share their story, followed by 2 minutes of group feedback. Be sure to keep track of time so that each person has enough time to share and receive feedback.

HEALTHY RELATIONSHIPS
WHAT IS SECURE ATTACHMENT ?

> Before the groups begin sharing, it is a good idea to ask participants to raise their hands if they get stuck, have questions or need help once small group sharing begins. Be ready to help as needed.
>
> You will need to keep careful track of time in this exercise.

1. This exercise will help you learn to tell a Level 4+ story about secure attachment.

2. Locate your Level 4+ Secure Attachment Story Worksheet that is in your workbook. Your facilitator will take 5 minutes to review the worksheet and characteristics of a Level 4+ story with you.

3. To help you begin thinking about secure attachment, your facilitator will ask the question, "What do secure attachments feel like?"
   a. Your facilitator will share a few words describing what secure attachments with God and others feel like to him/her.
   b. Your facilitator will ask volunteers to share one word describing what secure attachments with God and others feel like.
   c. You will have 3 minutes for this part of the exercise, and your facilitator will keep track of time for you.

4. Your facilitator will share a Level 4+ Secure Attachment Story with you. After the story, your facilitator will ask the group for feedback. Did his/her story include all the characteristics listed on the worksheet? You will have 5 minutes for this part of the exercise. Your facilitator will keep track of time for you.

5. Break into groups of 3 people.

6. Take 5 minutes to complete the "Preparing My Level 4+ Secure Attachment Story" worksheet that is in your workbook. For this exercise:
   a. If you have ever had a relationship with a person who has a secure attachment style, describe a specific experience that you had with them.
   b. If you have never had a relationship with a person who has a secure attachment style, you may describe a time in which you experienced secure attachment in your relationship with God.
   c. If you have had no experience with secure attachments, imagine what a secure attachment might feel like. Complete your worksheet, and describe what kind of securely attached relationship you would like to have. How do you think it might feel? How do you think you would like to act in a secure relationship? Have you ever seen a securely attached relationship between others?
   d. Your facilitator will help you know when it is time to begin telling stories.

7. Your facilitator will ask for volunteers in each small group to begin telling a Level 4+ Secure Attachment Story. You will have 3 minutes to tell your story. Your facilitator will keep track of time for you. If at any point your group is stuck or has a question, please raise your hand, and your facilitator will come help you.

8. After the first secure attachment story, each group can take 2 minutes to give feedback on the story. Use the "Preparing My Level 4+ Secure Attachment Story" worksheet as a guideline to help the storyteller discover if he/she was able to share all the elements of a 4+ story that are listed on the worksheet. Be encouraging and positive! Your facilitator will keep track of time for you, and let you know when it is time for the next person to share his/her story.

YOUR NOTES

HEALTHY RELATIONSHIPS
WHAT IS SECURE ATTACHMENT?

YOUR NOTES

9. Your facilitator will let you know when it is time for a second person in each small group to begin his/her 3-minute Level 4+ Secure Attachment Story, followed by 2 minutes of feedback. Your facilitator will keep track of time for you and let you know when it is time for the next person to share his/her story.

10. Your facilitator will let you know when it is time for the third person in each small group to begin his/her 3-minute Level 4+ Secure Attachment Story, followed by 2 minutes of feedback. Your facilitator will keep track of time for you.

11. At the conclusion of the exercise, participants may remain in their small groups. If time permits, your facilitator will ask volunteers to share about their experiences with the entire group. Use one word to describe how it felt to share and hear stories about secure attachment.

CLOSE THE GROUP WITH PRAYER

HEALTHY RELATIONSHIPS
WHAT IS SECURE ATTACHMENT ?

QUESTIONS FOR FURTHER DISCUSSION OR FOLLOW-UP

1. What does "Secure Attachment" mean to you?

2. Do you think that anything you have done keeps God from wanting secure attachment with you? Why?

3. Have you ever avoided God because you felt ashamed of BEEPS – or didn't feel "good enough" to attach to Him? What made you this way?

4. Have you ever felt like you had to "clean up" or "behave" so that God would be happy to be with you? What did you do to try to improve yourself? Did it work?

5. What does Revelation 3:20 mean to you?

6. Why do you need secure attachment to be fulfilled?

7. What do you think life would be like if you could bring and give life wherever you go?

8. How would you describe attachment pain? What is it?

9. Why does attachment pain make good solutions turn sour or sexual? Has this ever happened to you?

10. Why is it important for you to learn to recognize attachment pain?

11. Have you ever tried a "quick fix" for attachment pain? Describe the pain – and what happened when you tried the "quick fix."

12. Have you ever tried to use God or religious experience as a "quick fix" for attachment pain? What happened?

13. What BEEPS have you used to medicate or relieve attachment pain? Use the list below to mark the BEEPS that you've used in attachment pain. Did any of these work?

- [ ] Alcohol
- [ ] Other Drugs
- [ ] Relationships
- [ ] Sex
- [ ] Food
- [ ] Gambling
- [ ] Work
- [ ] Performance/Perfectionism
- [ ] Thrill-seeking Behaviors
- [ ] Computer
- [ ] Video Games
- [ ] TV
- [ ] Money
- [ ] Power and Control
- [ ] Internet or Internet Pornography
- [ ] Religion or Ministry
- [ ] Cutting
- [ ] Rage
- [ ] Other: Be Specific

HEALTHY RELATIONSHIPS
WHAT IS SECURE ATTACHMENT ?

QUESTIONS FOR FURTHER DISCUSSION OR FOLLOW-UP

14. Have BEEPS brought you to a place of absolute powerlessness, absolute unmanageability and absolute insanity? Why – or why not?

15. What does it mean to "turn your will and life" over to the care of God?

16. Who is God – and who do you understand God to be? Draw a picture illustrating your concept of God – and your relationship to Him.

17. What did you learn from the Level 4+ secure attachment stories?

OPTIONAL 12-STEP QUESTIONS

1. What BEEPS have you used to medicate or relieve attachment pain? Use the list below to mark the BEEPS that you've used in attachment pain. Did any of these work?

   - [ ] Alcohol
   - [ ] Other Drugs
   - [ ] Relationships
   - [ ] Sex
   - [ ] Food
   - [ ] Gambling
   - [ ] Work
   - [ ] Performance/Perfectionism
   - [ ] Thrill-seeking Behaviors
   - [ ] Computer
   - [ ] Video Games
   - [ ] TV
   - [ ] Money
   - [ ] Power and Control
   - [ ] Internet or Internet Pornography
   - [ ] Religion or Ministry
   - [ ] Cutting
   - [ ] Rage
   - [ ] Other: Be Specific

2. Does attachment pain make your life unmanageable? Does it leave you feeling powerless?

3. Insanity can be described as "doing the same thing over and over again, and always expecting a different result. Does medicating attachment pain with BEEPS fit this definition of insanity?

4. What is Step 3? Describe it in your own words.

5. What does it mean to turn your will over to the care of God? What does it mean to you?

6. What does it mean to turn your life over to the care of God? What does it mean to you?

7. What did you learn and believe about God growing up?

HEALTHY RELATIONSHIPS
WHAT IS SECURE ATTACHMENT ?

OPTIONAL 12-STEP QUESTIONS

8. Who had the most influence on your concept of God when you were a child? Was there a difference between what they said about God – and how they lived? How did this affect you?

9. What did your concept of God look like when you were a child? What kind of attachment did you have with Him? Draw a picture that illustrates your concept of God at that time in your life– and your attachment with Him.

10. What kind of choices did you make about your attachment with God when you were old enough to make them for yourself?

11. Has your use of BEEPS ever affected your attachment with God? Draw a picture that illustrates how BEEPS have affected this relationship.

12. What do you believe about God at this point in your life? What do you think God is like? What kind of relationship would you like to have with God now?

13. What is your attachment with God at this time? Draw a picture that illustrates your attachment with Him at this point in your life.

14. Do you think God cares about your life? How would you like Him to help you?

15. What do you believe about Jesus? Do you think that He is willing to help you if you ask?

16. Are you afraid that you will be disappointed if you ask Jesus to help you?

17. Is there anybody in your life that could help you grow in your understanding of God? Who are they? Are you willing to ask them to help you?

18. Making a decision is a very left-brained logical process. Attachment is a right brain process that involves relationship and experience with the person we want to attach to.
    a. What do you think would happen if you asked Jesus if He was willing to help you? Would you like to ask Him for help?
    b. Take a moment and ask Him this question, "Jesus, are you willing to help me?"
    c. Wait quietly for a few minutes, and pay attention to any impression, experience or perception that you may have.
    d. Write down any impression, experience or perceptions that you may have.
    e. Ask the person that you've identified in question 17 to help you understand this experience.

PREPARING MY 4+ SECURE ATTACHMENT STORY WORKSHEET

1. This story has a moderate feeling level and is not too intense ☐

2. I have told this story before ☐

3. I do not need to be guarded in telling this story ☐

4. This story is autobiographical (I am involved in the story) ☐

5. This story illustrates a specific feeling ☐

6. I will show the authentic emotion on my face and in my voice ☐

7. I will maintain eye contact while storytelling ☐

8. Briefly describe the situation:

9. Feeling words for this story:

10. During this story my body felt:

11. The things I did in this story that demonstrate how I like to act in this emotion are (or if I did not act like myself at the time, it would have been like me to do this…)

6 PAINFUL RELATIONSHIPS
DISMISSIVE AND DISTRACTED ATTACHMENT

OPEN THE GROUP

- Ask for a volunteer to open the group in prayer.

EXERCISE: ATTACHMENT PAIN SONGS *5 Minutes*

Facilitator Note: This exercise helps participants review the concept of attachment pain they learned last week. It is also a fun way to start group and facilitate participation.

In this exercise, your group will share examples of songs with themes of attachment pain that they heard – or thought of – in the past week. They can also share about any songs that were discussed in last week's attachment pain and popular music exercise. When volunteers have finished sharing, the group can vote on their favorite attachment pain song. Have fun with this exercise!

It is helpful to prepare for this exercise by finding a few examples of songs with themes of attachment pain that you can share at the beginning of this exercise.

1. This exercise helps review the concept of attachment pain as it is expressed in popular music. In this exercise, your group will vote to determine its favorite attachment pain song.

2. Your facilitator will share one or two songs with a theme of attachment pain.

3. Your facilitator will ask volunteers to share about an attachment pain song they heard in the past week – or one they have thought about since the last session.

4. Ask the group to pay attention to the songs that volunteers share.

5. When the last volunteer has shared, the group can vote (raise their hands) to decide which song best describes attachment pain.

TODAY'S LESSON: Dismissive and Distracted Attachment

Facilitator Note: Play Session Six on the Restarting DVD.
- Ask the class to follow along in their workbooks, and take notes as needed.
- Please note that you will need to stop the video several times to lead exercises. The video will let you know when to stop.

CLASS NOTES: Dismissive and Distracted Attachment

There are four attachment styles
- Secure
- Dismissive

PAINFUL RELATIONSHIPS
DISMISSIVE AND DISTRACTED ATTACHMENT

- Distracted
- Disorganized

Secure attachment results from high joy capacity and synchronized bonds.
- How do non-secure attachments form?

Non-secure attachments result from:
- Lack of joy capacity.
- Lack of synchronization.
- Getting stuck in pain without the ability to return to joy.
- These keep us further disconnected from joyful relationships with God and others.

What happened to separate us?
- Even when we want our relationships to work?
- Why do relationships hurt so much?

After the Fall:
- Then the eyes of both of them were opened, and they knew that they were naked; and they sewed fig leaves together and made themselves coverings. And they heard the sound of the Lord God walking in the garden in the cool of the day, and Adam and his wife hid themselves from the presence of the Lord God among the trees of the garden. Then the Lord God called to Adam and said to him, "Where are you?" So he said, "I heard Your voice in the garden, and I was afraid because I was naked; and I hid myself." And He said, "Who told you that you were naked? Have you eaten from the tree of which I commanded you that you should not eat?" Then the man said, "The woman whom You gave to be with me, she gave me of the tree, and I ate." And the Lord God said to the woman, "What is this you have done?" The woman said, "The serpent deceived me, and I ate." Genesis 3:7-10. NKJV.

Fear

Shame

Covering up

Hiding and denial

Blaming and accusing

Anger
- To Adam he said, "Cursed is the ground because of you; through painful toil you will eat of it all the days of your life. It will produce thorns and thistles for you, and you will eat the plants of the field. By the sweat of your brow (your sweaty, angry, red face) you will eat your food until you return to the ground, since from dust you were taken; for dust you are and to dust you will return. Gen. 3: 17-19, NIV, (parenthesis and highlight added).

Sadness
- To the Woman he said, "I will greatly increase your pains (sorrows) in childbearing; with pain you will give birth to children. Your desire will be for your husband, and he will rule over you. Gen. 3:16 NIV, (parenthesis and highlight added).

PAINFUL RELATIONSHIPS
DISMISSIVE AND DISTRACTED ATTACHMENT

YOUR NOTES

Relationships – that were designed to be a source of strength and joy – became a source of pain.
- Lack of synchronization, diminished capacity and pain drive insecure attachments.

Non-secure attachments can lead to pain at any level of the control center.
- Level 1: Attachment pain
- Level 2: Pervasive fear
- Level 3: Desynchronized, stuck in negative emotions
- Level 4: Immaturity
- Level 5: Inconsistent identity

Dismissive attachment

Dismissive
- Parent/caregiver not available.
- Detached and not synchronized to child needs for attachment on a regular basis.
- I can't expect connection, so I will live life on my own.
- Low affect, rejection, anger.
- Virtual Other: uncaring, unavailable.

Attachment light: Off
- The control center is underdeveloped.
- Life is painful – but less painful than having no one to attach to me.
- It is stuck in a parasympathetic dominant state of response to people and relationships.
- Copes through energy-conservation state of withdrawal.
- Has problems shifting out of low arousal states into intense negative or positive affect.

Adult relationships:
- Distant and avoidant.
- Withdrawal as coping strategy.
- May be highly competent or workaholic – but will operate from duty – not joy.
- Can't synchronize or share mutual mind.
- Dismisses the importance of emotions and relationships.
- Life is safer – and feels better alone and undisturbed.

What does dismissive attachment look like?
- Pause for a Level 4 Dismissive Attachment Story

EXERCISE: TELLING A LEVEL 4 DISMISSIVE ATTACHMENT STORY
10 Minutes.

> **Facilitator Note:** Please stop the video at this point for the exercise.
>
> This exercise is designed to help participants identify and understand dismissive attachment by telling non-verbal stories. Volunteers will answer the question, "What does dismissive attachment look like?" without using words.
> A word about Level 4 stories: In this Level 4 story exercise, participants tell their stories without using words. While Level 4+ stories combine elements of both the left hemis-

PAINFUL RELATIONSHIPS
DISMISSIVE AND DISTRACTED ATTACHMENT

phere (words) and right hemisphere (emotions) of the brain, Level 4 stories are different. In Level 4 stories, participants act out the story they are describing using facial expression, body language, and movement. This exercise allows the right hemisphere of the brain to express itself – without using words.

Level 4 stories are a lot of fun for groups. It may help to describe Level 4 stories as an opportunity to "Go to Hollywood," because it gives everyone a chance to try out their acting skills. The Level 4 Dismissive Attachment Exercise can be a lot of fun – and an excellent way to help participants understand dismissive attachment.

To lead this exercise, you will first need to explain Level 4 stories to your group. Next, prepare your group to tell their stories by helping them identify the behaviors and feelings they have associated with dismissive attachment. You can start this process by sharing one-word descriptions of what dismissive attachment is like – or what it feels like trying to relate to a person with dismissive attachment. Volunteers will also have the opportunity to do the same. Finally, you will need to demonstrate a Level 4 Dismissive Attachment Story for the entire group. The best way for them to learn how to tell a Level 4 story is by watching you!

Because Level 4 Dismissive Attachment Stories usually only last for a few seconds, you should be able to complete this exercise in 10 minutes.

1. For this exercise, it is not necessary to break into small groups.

2. Your facilitator will explain Level 4 stories.
   a. Level 4 stories are non-verbal stories that are told without using words.
   b. Level 4+ stories combine elements of both the left hemisphere (words) and right hemisphere (emotions) of the brain.
   c. Level 4 stories express the experiences, feelings, and sensations of the right hemisphere, without using words from the left hemisphere of the brain to describe them.
   d. In Level 4 stories, participants act-out the story and emotions they are describing using only facial expression, body language, movement or non-verbal interactions with others.

3. To begin the exercise:
   a. Your facilitator will begin the exercise by asking the group if they have ever known anyone who has a dismissive attachment style.
   b. Your facilitator will share one-word descriptions of what dismissive attachment is like – or what it feels like relating to a person with dismissive attachment.
   c. Volunteers may share one-word descriptions of what dismissive attachment is like – or what it feels like trying to relate to a person with dismissive attachment.

4. Your facilitator will tell a Level 4 Dismissive Attachment Story for the entire group that describes what dismissive attachment looks like.

5. Volunteers have the opportunity to tell a Level 4 Dismissive Attachment Story that answers the question, "What does dismissive attachment look like?" Remember to tell these stories using only facial expression, body language, movement or non-verbal interactions with others. Have fun with this! You are "Going Hollywood."

6. Your facilitator will keep track of time for you, and will let you know when it is time to restart the video.

Facilitator Note: Restart the video.

PAINFUL RELATIONSHIPS
DISMISSIVE AND DISTRACTED ATTACHMENT

YOUR NOTES

Distracted attachment

Distracted
- Parent sends mixed signals about attachment.
- Interactions tend to be intrusive and are based on parent – not infant state of mind.
- Infant needs sometimes met, sometimes unmet – never knows which.
- Child becomes preoccupied with attachment.

The attachment light: Always On
- It is stuck in a sympathetic dominant state of response to people and relationships.
- High emotions, without ability to quiet self.
- Fear and anger are high arousal states without ability to regulate.
- Impulsive and excitable, little capacity for stress.
- It is hard to live life when always distracted by the possibility of attaching to someone – or something!

Adult relationships:
- Highly needy, dependent and anxious - focused on receiving comfort for distress.
- Can quickly "attach" in high energy relationships – and appear quite functional – and then overwhelm others.
- Frequent highly emotional displays.
- Can use "neediness" or distress to manipulate others for attention.
- One crisis after another.

What does distracted attachment look like?
- Pause for a Level 4 Distracted Attachment Story.

EXERCISE: TELLING A LEVEL 4 DISTRACTED ATTACHMENT STORY
10 Minutes.

> **Facilitator Note:** Please stop the video at this point for the exercise.
>
> This exercise is designed to help participants identify and understand dismissive attachment by telling non-verbal stories. Volunteers will answer the question, "What does dismissive attachment look like?" without using words.
>
> It is helpful to begin this exercise by reminding participants that Level 4 stories are told without words, using start facial expression, body language, and movement. Next, prepare your group to tell their stories by helping them identify the behaviors and feelings they have associated with distracted attachment. You can start this process by sharing one-word descriptions of what distracted attachment is like – or what it feelings like trying to relate to a person with distracted attachment. You can then invite volunteers to do the same. Finally, you will need to demonstrate a Level 4 Distracted Attachment Story for the entire group. The best way for them to learn how to tell a Level 4 story is by watching you!
>
> Level 4 stories are a lot of fun for groups. It may help to describe Level 4 stories as an opportunity to "Go to Hollywood," because it gives everyone a chance to try out their acting skills. This Level 4 Distracted Attachment Exercise can be a lot of fun – and an

PAINFUL RELATIONSHIPS
DISMISSIVE AND DISTRACTED ATTACHMENT

> excellent way to help participants understand distracted attachment.
>
> Because Level 4 Distracted Attachment Stories usually only last for a few seconds, you should be able to complete this exercise in 10 minutes.

1. For this exercise, it is not necessary to break into small groups.

2. Your facilitator will remind you that Level 4 stories are non-verbal, and are told using facial expressions, body language and movement.

3. To begin the exercise:
   a. Your facilitator will begin the exercise by asking the group if they have ever known anyone who has a distracted attachment style.
   b. Your facilitator will share one-word description of what distracted attachment is like – or what it feels like trying to relate to a person with distracted attachment.
   c. Volunteers may share one-word descriptions of what distracted attachment is like – or what it feels like trying to relate to a person with distracted attachment.

4. Your facilitator will tell a Level 4 Distracted Attachment Story for the entire group that describes what distracted attachment looks like.

5. Volunteers have the opportunity to tell Level 4 Distracted Attachment Story that answers the question, "What does distracted attachment look like?" Remember to tell these stories using only facial expression, body language, movement or non-verbal interactions with others. Have fun with this! You are "Going Hollywood."

6. Your facilitator will keep track of time for you, and will let you know when it is time to restart the video.

Facilitator Note: Restart the video.

Non-secure attachment is painful.
- Our level of pain is higher than our level of joy.
- This is experienced as trauma and ongoing relational distress.
- But it gets worse!

Non-secure attachment will continue to traumatize and reduce capacity.
- Non-secure attachments lead to a level of pain that exceeds our joy capacity, and this means that we tend to live in ongoing trauma and distress.
- Non-secure attachments continue to make the problem worse because they cause increasing levels of pain and distress – and decrease our levels of joy.
- Our level of trauma worsens.
- We are continually re-traumatized by our non-secure attachments.

Medicate to regulate

BEEPS
- BEEPS are attachments to Behaviors, Events, Experiences, People or Substances that are used to regulate emotions, increase pleasure or decrease pain.

BEEPS
- Attachments to BEEPS help us medicate – to artificially regulate – positive and

PAINFUL RELATIONSHIPS
DISMISSIVE AND DISTRACTED ATTACHMENT

negative emotions as well as pain.

BEEPS
- Attachments to BEEPS take the place of secure attachments to God and significant others.

BEEPS
- There are many different types of BEEPS. Examples can include:
- Behaviors: Work
- Events: Thrill Seeking
- Experiences: Sex
- People: Relationships
- Substances: Alcohol

Step 4: made a fearless and searching moral inventory of ourselves.

Taking a fearless and searching look at myself.
- Step 4 can only happen when we have attached ourselves to a Power greater than ourselves – someone who is empowered by joy and is genuinely glad to be with us!
- Step 4 is not just about BEEPS.
- Step 4 is about:
  - Identifying the issues and pain that led to BEEPS.
  - Recognizing what my attachments to BEEPS did to my life and relationships.
- Unless I identify the problem and take steps to correct it, I will repeat it!

Step 5: Admitted to God, to ourselves and to another human being the exact nature of our wrongs.

Getting honest with God, myself and others who are empowered by joy and are willing to share my distress:
- Breaks Isolation.
- Helps break attachments to BEEPS by helping me attach to others.
- Helps build secure, joyful bonds!

Attachment style can become more secure and joyful!

EXERCISE: LEVEL 4+ RETURNING TO JOY FROM NEGATIVE EMOTIONS
STORY *30 Minutes*

Facilitator Note: The purpose of this exercise is to help participants learn to tell a Level 4+ story about an experience in which they were able to return to joy from one of the Big Six negative emotions.

As you recall, Level 4+ stories help build joy and capacity. They can also provide us with examples of how other people act – or like to act – while they are experiencing different emotions. Level 4+ stories are powerful, because they involve all four levels of the emotional control center in the right hemisphere of the brain – plus the verbal left hemisphere. Level 4+ Return to Joy from Negative Emotions Stories provide vivid illustrations of how others have experienced negative emotions – and been able to return to joy. Hearing these stories helps participants learn from each other and improve their capacity to return to joy from negative emotions.

YOUR NOTES

PAINFUL RELATIONSHIPS
DISMISSIVE AND DISTRACTED ATTACHMENT

In previous weeks, participants have practiced telling Level 4+ stories about experiences with joy and secure attachment. In this week's exercise, participants will learn to tell a Level 4+ story about a time when they experienced one of the Big Six negative emotions, and were able to return to joy. In Weeks 3 and 4, we learned that the Big Six negative emotions are anger, fear, sadness, shame, disgust and hopeless despair. For this exercise, participants can tell their story about a time when they returned to joy from anger, fear or sadness.

You may find it helpful to review the facilitator notes and instructions for Level 4+ stories in Chapter 4 and Chapter 5 as you prepare for this exercise. It is also a good idea to go over the characteristics of a Level 4+ story listed on your "Preparing My Level 4+ Return to Joy Story Worksheet." Since you will be telling a Level 4+ Return to Joy Story for participants, be sure to complete your worksheet and practice your story ahead of time. Be aware that there is a significant difference between this exercise and previous Level 4+ story exercises. While previous Level 4+ stories focused exclusively on positive experiences and joyful emotions, this exercise focuses on returning to joy from the negative emotions of anger, fear or sadness.

Remember, to the brain, joy means relationship. It means, "Someone is glad to be with me!" As we learn to "Return to Joy," we are discovering how to act like the person God has created us to be – and stay relational with others – when we experience a negative emotion. Returning to joy is about learning to act like ourselves so that we stay connected to others when we are distressed.

To help participants prepare to tell their Level 4+ Return to Joy Story, make sure they locate the "Preparing My Level 4+ Return to Joy Story Worksheet," in their workbook. Ask them to follow along with you as you review the elements of a Level 4+ Return to Joy Story. Make sure they understand that as they complete the worksheet, they will need to describe a situation in which they felt the emotion of anger, fear, or sadness, list feeling words to describe the emotion, and describe how their body felt when they experienced the negative emotion. Because this is a story involving negative emotions, it is a good idea to remind everyone to make sure that the story is of moderate intensity, and that it is a story they do not need to be guarded in telling.

It is also helpful to clarify the questions, "What did I do in the story that demonstrates how I like to act when I am this upset? What did I do that helped me return to joy? If I wasn't able to return to joy – or didn't act like me when I was upset – what would I have liked to do?"

These questions are an important part of Return to Joy stories, since it is likely that some participants will describe an experience in which they were unable to return to joy – or did not act like themselves when they were upset. The questions help these participants by asking them to describe, identify and understand how they truly like to act – or want to act – when they experience a distressing negative emotion. This helps them answer the essential question, "What is it really like me to do when I am this upset?" This can help them develop new strategies for dealing with negative emotions.

When you have finished reviewing the worksheet, tell your own Return to Joy from Negative Emotions Story! The best way for participants to learn to tell this type of Level 4+ story is to hear one. Limit your story to 3 minutes.

After you have finished your story, ask your group for 2 minutes of feedback to help you determine if your story met all the guidelines for Level 4+ stories listed on the worksheet. Read each characteristic listed on the worksheet, and then ask your group if your Level 4+ story met each one. Remind your group that feedback on Level 4+ stories does

PAINFUL RELATIONSHIPS
DISMISSIVE AND DISTRACTED ATTACHMENT

> not include comments, criticisms or advice based on the experience or feelings shared during a story. Feedback is based solely on the worksheet guidelines.
>
> When feedback is complete, it is time for participants to take 5 minutes and complete their own "Preparing My Level 4+ Return to Joy Story Worksheet." When they are finished, volunteers may begin sharing their stories with their small group. Volunteers will have 3 minutes to share their story, followed by 2 minutes of group feedback. Be sure to keep track of time so that each person has enough time to share and receive feedback.
>
> Before the groups begin sharing, it is a good idea to ask participants to raise their hands if they get stuck, have questions or need help once small group sharing begins. Be ready to help as needed.

YOUR NOTES

1. This exercise will help you learn to tell a Level 4+ Return to Joy from Negative Emotions Story.
   a. Your story should describe a time when you experienced the emotion of anger ear or sadness – and were able to return to joy afterwards.
   b. If you can't remember a time when you experienced these negative emotions and were able to return to joy, explain what you now think you might have been able to do to help you return to joy in the situation you've described. You can also explain how you would like to act in a similar situation that might help you return to joy.
   c. Remember, to the brain, joy means relationship. It means, "Someone is glad to be with me!" As we learn to "Return to Joy," we are discovering how to act like the person God has created us to be – and stay relational with others – when we experience a negative emotion. Returning to joy is about learning to act like ourselves so that we stay connected to others when we are distressed.

2. Locate your "Preparing My Level 4+ Return to Joy Story Worksheet" in your workbook. Your facilitator will take 5 minutes to review the worksheet and characteristics of a Level 4+ Return to Joy from Negative Emotions Story with you. Because this is a story that describes an experience in which you experienced a negative emotion, pay particular attention to the following:
   a. Make sure your story is of moderate intensity so others are not overwhelmed.
   b. Make sure this is a story that you don't need to be guarded in telling.

3. To describe the experience, emotions, body sensations and what you did when you were upset:
   a. Describe the situation. What was occurring when you felt anger, fear or sadness?
   b. List feeling words to describe what anger, fear or sadness felt like to you.
   c. Describe the sensations you felt in your body when you were upset. What was going on in your body?
   d. What did you do in the story that demonstrates how you like to act when you feel anger, fear or sadness? What did you do in your story that illustrates how you "acted like you" when you were upset?
   e. What did you do to return to joy?
   f. If you were unable to return to joy in the situation you described, how do you now think you might have been able to "act like yourself" and return to joy? How would you like to act in a similar situation and return to joy? This is helping you answer the question, "What is it like me to do when I am this upset?" How can "acting like you" help you return to joy in the future?

4. Your facilitator will share a 3-minute Level 4+ Return to Joy story with you.

PAINFUL RELATIONSHIPS
DISMISSIVE AND DISTRACTED ATTACHMENT

5. You will have 2 minutes to give your facilitator feedback on his/her story.
   a. Your facilitator will read each element listed on the worksheet, and ask volunteers to help determine if the story contained each element.
   b. Feedback is designed to help a storyteller determine if the story contained each element listed on the worksheet. It should not include criticism or advice about the experience or emotions described in the story.

6. Break into groups of 3 people.

7. Take 5 minutes to complete the "Preparing My Level 4+ Return to Joy Story Worksheet." You may describe a situation in which you experienced an emotion of anger, fear or sadness. Your facilitator will keep track of time for you.

8. Your facilitator will ask for volunteers in each small group to begin telling a Level 4+ Return to Joy Story. You will have 3 minutes to tell your story. Your facilitator will keep track of time for you. If at any point your group is stuck or has a question, please raise your hand, and your facilitator will come help you.

9. After the first joy story, each group can take 2 minutes to give feedback on the story. Use the "Preparing My Level 4+ Return to Joy Story Worksheet" as a guideline to help the storyteller discover if they were able to share all the elements of a 4+ story that are listed on the worksheet. Be encouraging and positive! Your facilitator will keep track of time for you, and let you know when it is time for the next person to share their story.

10. Your facilitator will let you know when it is time for a second person in each small group to begin their 3-minute Level 4+ Return to Joy Story, followed by 2 minutes of feedback. Your facilitator will keep track of time for you and let you know when it is time for the next person to share their story.

11. Your facilitator will let you know when it is time for the third person in each small group to begin their 3-minute Level 4+ Return to Joy Story, followed by 2 minutes of feedback. Your facilitator will keep track of time for you.

12. At the conclusion of the exercise, participants may remain in their small groups. If time permits, your facilitator will ask volunteers to share about their experience with the entire group. Use one word to describe how it felt to share these stories.

OPTIONAL EXERCISES

EXERCISE: RUNNING TO STAND STILL *25 Minutes*

Facilitator Note: In this exercise, you will use a song about a heroin user to help participants explore the connection between BEEPS – and the people who use BEEPS. The goal of this exercise is to help participants apply the information they've learned about non-secure attachments to both BEEPS, and the relational trauma that results from attachments to BEEPS.

For this exercise, you will need a copy of the song "Running to Stand Still" by U2 from their CD "The Joshua Tree." Due to copyright and licensing restrictions, we cannot provide you with a copy of the song.

PAINFUL RELATIONSHIPS
DISMISSIVE AND DISTRACTED ATTACHMENT

> You can obtain a copy of "The Joshua Tree" CD through online vendors or stores where CDs are sold. The song "Running to Stand Still" may also be purchased and downloaded separately through online music vendors.
>
> The song is also available in video format from concert footage on "Rattle and Hum" or "Zoo TV Live from Sydney." If you would prefer to use the video version of this song, "Rattle and Hum" and "Zoo TV Live from Sydney" are widely available at CD/Video outlets, online vendors or www.U2.com.
>
> If you do not wish to use the song in either audio or video format, you may read participants the words to the song, which are available online. Please check online resources including www.U2.com.
>
> If you choose the video format, you will need either a VCR or DVD – and TV for this exercise. If you use the CD or downloaded version of the song, make sure that you have the appropriate music player and speakers available for your group.
>
> Be sure that you preview this song before you lead this exercise.

YOUR NOTES

1. Break into small groups of 3-5 people.

2. In this exercise, you will be using the song "Running to Stand Still," which is about a person who is using heroin. The goal of this exercise is to help you apply the information you've learned about non-secure attachments to both BEEPS, and to the relational trauma that results from attachments to BEEPS.

3. Your facilitator may share this song with you in audio or video format – or may read the song lyrics to you.

4. As you listen to the song, pay attention to:
   a. The relationship the woman in the song has with heroin.
   b. The relationship the woman in the story has to the person who is telling the story.

5. When the song is finished, you will have 15 minutes to share the answers to these questions with your group:
   a. How did the woman's attachment to heroin affect her?
   b. How do you think the woman's use of heroin affected her relationship with the person telling the story? Was her attachment with this person secure or non-secure? Why?
   c. Your facilitator will help you by keeping track of time.

6. After 15 minutes of sharing, you may remain in your groups, and your facilitator will lead you in a short relaxation exercise.

EXERCISE: LEARNING TO BREATHE DEEPLY *2 Minutes*

> **Facilitator Note:** This exercise helps participants practice relaxation skills they first learned in Week 2. In this exercise, participants learn to relax as they breathe deeply and share "Quiet Together" time.

PAINFUL RELATIONSHIPS
DISMISSIVE AND DISTRACTED ATTACHMENT

YOUR NOTES

1. Follow your facilitator's instructions as you do this exercise.

2. Remain in your small groups. Stand up, and make sure that you have 3-4 feet of clear space around you.

3. Imagine that you are a marionette – a puppet – with a string running from the base of your spine to the top of your head. Imagine that the string is gently pulled upwards and your back, neck and head are perfectly aligned. Your head is at rest and comfortably settled in line with your back and spine. You are looking forward, and your head is settled in comfortably.

4. Bend your knees slightly. You are standing still in a comfortable position.

5. Place your hand over your stomach.

6. Take such a deep breath that you feel your stomach expand as you breathe. Follow your facilitator's instructions as you breathe deeply for a few moments.

7. Your facilitator will keep track of time for you as you relax and breathe deeply and relax.

CLOSE THE GROUP WITH PRAYER

PAINFUL RELATIONSHIPS
DISMISSIVE AND DISTRACTED ATTACHMENT

QUESTIONS FOR FURTHER DISCUSSION OR FOLLOW-UP

1. How do non-secure attachments form?

2. How would you describe the attachment Adam, Eve and God shared before the fall?

3. What happened to Adam and Eve's attachment with God after the fall?

4. As a result of the fall, Adam and Eve began to relate to God and each other through:
   a. Fear
   b. Shame
   c. Covering Up
   d. Hiding and Denial
   e. Blaming and Accusing
   f. Anger
   g. Sadness

   How have these negative emotions and behaviors each affected your relationship with God – and other relationships that are important to you? Be very specific.

5. Please list 5 characteristics of dismissive attachment.

6. Do you know someone (including yourself) who has dismissive attachment? How does this attachment style make it difficult to develop secure attachments? Be specific.

7. From what you learned in this week's lesson, how does a person with dismissive attachment typically deal with conflict?

8. Why might a person with dismissive attachment tend to develop a BEEPS with work?

9. Please list 5 characteristics of distracted attachment.

10. Do you know someone (including yourself) who has distracted attachment? How does this attachment style make it difficult to develop secure attachments? Be specific.

11. From what you learned in this week's lesson, how does a person with distracted attachment typically deal with conflict?

12. Why might a person with dismissive attachment tend to develop a BEEPS with relationships?

13. Why do non-secure attachments lead to more trauma and distress in relationships?

14. Why is it important to identify issues of pain, attachment and BEEPS in our lives?

15. How does "getting honest" about our pain, attachments and BEEPS with someone else who is empowered by joy help us in our recovery?

16. What did you learn from the "Running to Stand Still" Exercise?

PAINFUL RELATIONSHIPS
DISMISSIVE AND DISTRACTED ATTACHMENT

OPTIONAL 12-STEP QUESTIONS

1. How did you feel during the "Running to Stand Still" exercise? Has your use of BEEPS caused your life to stand still – or have your attachments to BEEPS taken you backwards? Who did you identify with more in the song: The heroin user – or the person in relationship with them?

2. Which of these emotions and behaviors discussed in this week's lesson have been difficult for you?
   - Fear
   - Shame
   - Covering Up
   - Hiding and Denial
   - Blaming and Accusing
   - Anger
   - Sadness

3. How have these affected your life and relationships with God and other people? Be specific.

4. Have you ever used BEEPS to deal with these negative emotions and behaviors? Which BEEPS have you used to help you with these feelings and behaviors?

5. Do you think that your own non-secure attachments have caused you pain? What kind of pain did you experience? How long have you had this pain?

6. Do you have a dismissive or distracted attachment style? How has this affected your life, relationships and attachments to BEEPS?

7. Did your mom, dad or the person who took care of you when you were growing up have dismissive or distracted attachments?

8. What do you expect from other people? How do you expect them to act and behave towards you? When did you learn to expect these things from others?

9. How long have you lived in the pain of non-secure attachment? Can you remember a time when you did not feel the pain of non-secure attachments?

10. Have you ever violated your own values through your use of BEEPS? Be specific. How did it happen – and did you feel guilty about it later? Do you continue to violate your own values with BEEPS today? How do you resolve – or medicate – your feelings of guilt about this?

11. When we are attached to BEEPS, we lose things that are important to us. How has your use of BEEPS caused you loss in these areas? Be specific.
    a. Relationships
    b. Work
    c. Opportunities
    d. Health
    e. Finances
    f. Possessions

12. When we are growing in our attachments with BEEPS, we tend to deny that we have a problem with BEEPS. We also tend to blame the problems BEEPS causes – that are too big to deny - on other people, places and things. Make a list of all the excuses that you've used to justify your use of BEEPS. Make a second list of all of the people, places and things that you've blamed for the problems BEEPS have caused.

13. When we've blamed other people, places and things for our problems, it is easy to develop resentments towards them. Make a list of the people that you've resented – for the problems BEEPS have caused you.

PAINFUL RELATIONSHIPS
DISMISSIVE AND DISTRACTED ATTACHMENT

OPTIONAL 12-STEP QUESTIONS

14. What is the worst moment of your attachment with BEEPS that you can remember? Describe it in detail.

15. How can admitting to God, yourself and another human being the pain and problems you've inventoried in these questions help your recovery?

16. Why is it important that the person you share these problems with be empowered by joy – and willing to share your distress? How can that help you?

17. Do you know anybody who is empowered by joy, and would be willing to share your distress? Who are they? What do you think would happen if you shared the pain and problems you've identified with them?

PREPARING MY 4+ RETURN TO JOY STORY WORKSHEET

1. This story has a moderate feeling level and is not too intense ☐

2. I have told this story before ☐

3. I do not need to be guarded in telling this story ☐

4. This story is autobiographical (I am involved in the story) ☐

5. This story illustrates a specific feeling ☐

6. I will show the authentic emotion on my face and in my voice ☐

7. I will maintain eye contact while storytelling ☐

8. Briefly describe the situation:

9. Feeling words for this story:

10. During this story my body felt:

11. The things I did in this story that demonstrate how I like to act in this emotion are (or if I did not act like myself at the time, it would have been like me to do this…)

7 TOXIC RELATIONSHIPS
DISORGANIZED ATTACHMENT AND TRAUMA

OPEN THE GROUP

- Ask for a volunteer to open the group in prayer.

EXERCISE: APPRECIATION EXERCISE *10 Minutes*

Facilitator Note: This is a joy and capacity building exercise that helps prepare participants for this week's lesson. As you lead this exercise, please remind participants to stay relational with each other as they share. To prepare for this exercise, it may be helpful to review the facilitator notes from Week 1.

1. Break into small groups of 3-5 people.

2. Your facilitator will ask each person to think about either:
   a. An experience they had with a person they especially appreciated in the past week.
   b. An experience they had with God this week that was especially meaningful.

3. Your facilitator will ask you each to take one minute to share with your group about the experience you had this week. Remember to:
   a. Maintain eye contact while sharing.
   b. Identify the person and experience that you appreciated
   c. Describe what emotions you felt during your experience.
   d. Describe what your body felt during that experience.

4. Your facilitator will help you by keeping track of time.
5. When each group is finished, your facilitator may ask volunteers to share how they feel after the exercise with the entire group. Use one or two words to describe your feelings.

TODAY'S LESSON: Disorganized Attachment and Trauma

Facilitator Note: Play Session Seven on the Restarting DVD.
- Ask the class to follow along in their workbooks, and take notes as needed.
- Please note that you will need to stop the video to lead an exercise. The video will let you know when to stop.

CLASS NOTES: Disorganized Attachment and Trauma

A quick review

YOUR NOTES

TOXIC RELATIONSHIPS
DISORGANIZED ATTACHMENT AND TRAUMA

There are four attachment styles:
- Secure
- Dismissive
- Distracted
- Disorganized

Secure attachment:
- Secure attachment results from high joy capacity and synchronized bonds.
- How do non-secure attachments form?

Non-secure attachments result from:
- Lack of joy capacity.
- Lack of synchronization.
- Getting stuck in pain without the ability to return to joy.
- These keep us further disconnected from joyful relationships with God and others.

After the Fall
- Then the eyes of both of them were opened, and they knew that they were naked; and they sewed fig leaves together and made themselves coverings And they heard the sound of the Lord God walking in the garden in the cool of the day, and Adam and his wife hid themselves from the presence of the Lord God among the trees of the garden. Then the Lord God called to Adam and said to him, "Where are you?" So he said, "I heard Your voice in the garden, and I was afraid because I was naked; and I hid myself." And He said, "Who told you that you were naked? Have you eaten from the tree of which I commanded you that you should not eat?" Then the man said, "The woman whom You gave to be with me, she gave me of the tree, and I ate." And the Lord God said to the woman, "What is this you have done?" The woman said, "The serpent deceived me, and I ate." Genesis 3:7-10. NKJV.

The relational consequences of the Fall include:
- Dismissive attachment.
- Distracted attachment.
- Disorganized attachment.

Disorganized attachment
- Relationship with parent/caregiver is the source of attachment and terror.
- Fear/terror of the attachment figure offers no comfort or synchronization – no soothing.
- Parent exhibits chaotic or disorganized behavior.
- Infant can't make sense of the "come here – go away" relationship.

Parent state
- Parents themselves have disorganized attachment, fear-based, dissociative, or disoriented behaviors.
- May include addictive behaviors.
- Physical, sexual, emotional abuse.
- 80% of abused children have disorganized attachment.

Adult relationships
- Highest likelihood of clinical problems.
- Hostile and aggressive with peers, controlling, difficult social relationships.
- Unregulated emotion followed by withdrawal.

TOXIC RELATIONSHIPS
DISORGANIZED ATTACHMENT AND TRAUMA

- Abusive patterns of behavior
- Virtual Other seen as important but terrifying, causing future relationships to fail, and increasing internal disorganization.
- Level 2 pain: pervasive fear and fear bonded relationships.

Domestic violence and disorganized attachment
- When the abuser feels needed – or asked to attach in any way – he or she is triggered into fear.
- The need could be anything from grocery money to affection.
- That fear may explode into rage – to make the pain stop and protect himself or herself.
- This pattern is highly likely if the abuser's spouse has distracted or disorganized attachment.
- You can't stop the violence by being a better wife, trying harder, not making him mad or "biblical submission."

Attachment and God
- Dismissive:
  - Avoidant and withdrawn
  - God at a distance, flat affect
- Distracted:
  - Anxious, needy
  - Performance and approval, high arousal, manipulative
- Disorganized:
  - Terror and fear
  - God is terrifying
  - Cults, spiritual abuse

The impacts of trauma and weak attachment on relationships
- Patterns of insecure or disorganized relationships continue throughout life, damaging relationships with friends, spouses and children.
- Series of ongoing unsatisfying relationships.
- Repeated relationship failures.
- Lack of joy-filled, mutually satisfying intimacy.
- Tend to over-react or withdraw from relationships.
- Overly dependent and needy or isolated and distant.
- Relationships are a source of pain – not comfort.
- Lack of mutual mind and synchronization.
- BEEPS

What does disorganized attachment look like?
- Pause for a Level 4 Disorganized Attachment Story.

EXERCISE: TELLING A LEVEL 4 DISORGANIZED ATTACHMENT STORY
10 Minutes

Facilitator Note: Please stop the video at this point for the exercise.

This exercise is designed to help participants identify and understand disorganized attachment by telling non-verbal stories. Volunteers will answer the question, "What does disorganized attachment look like?" without using words.

YOUR NOTES

TOXIC RELATIONSHIPS
DISORGANIZED ATTACHMENT AND TRAUMA

YOUR NOTES

As you learned last week, participants tell Level 4 stories without using words. While Level 4+ stories combine elements of both the left hemisphere (words) and right hemisphere (emotions) of the brain, Level 4 stories are different. In Level 4 stories, participants act out the story they are describing using facial expression, body language, and movement. This exercise allows the right hemisphere of the brain to express itself – without using words.

Level 4 stories are a lot of fun for groups. It may help to describe Level 4 stories as an opportunity to "Go to Hollywood," because it gives everyone a chance to try out their acting skills. The Level 4 Disorganized Attachment Exercise can be a lot of fun – and an excellent way to help participants understand disorganized attachment.

To lead this exercise, you will first need to review Level 4 stories to your group. Next, you can prepare your group to tell their stories by helping them identify the behaviors and feelings they have associated with disorganized attachment. You can start this process by sharing one-word descriptions of what disorganized attachment is like – or what it feels like trying to relate to a person with disorganized attachment. Volunteers will also have the opportunity to do the same. Finally, you will need to demonstrate a Level 4 Disorganized Attachment Story for the entire group. The best way for them to learn how to tell a Level 4 story is by watching you!

Because Level 4 Disorganized Attachment Stories usually only last for a few seconds, you should be able to complete this exercise in 10 minutes. Please be sensitive to the pain level in your group as you lead this exercise. Disorganized attachment is very painful, and you may shorten this exercise as needed.

1. For this exercise, it is not necessary to break into small groups.

2. Your facilitator will explain Level 4 stories.
   a. Level 4 stories are non-verbal stories that are told without using words.
   b. Level 4+ stories combine elements of both the left hemisphere (words) and right hemisphere (emotions) of the brain.
   c. Level 4 stories express the experiences, feelings, and sensations of the right hemisphere, without using words from the left hemisphere of the brain to describe them.
   d. In Level 4 stories, participants act out the story and emotions they are describing using only facial expression, body language, movement or non-verbal interactions with others.

3. To begin the exercise:
   a. Your facilitator will begin the exercise by asking the group if they have ever known anyone who has a disorganized attachment style.
   b. Your facilitator will share a one-word description of what disorganized attachment is like – or what it feels like trying to relate to a person with disorganized attachment.
   c. Volunteers share one-word descriptions of what disorganized attachment is like – or what it feels like trying to relate to a person with disorganized attachment.

4. Your facilitator will tell a Level 4 Disorganized Attachment Story for the entire group that describes what disorganized attachment looks like.

5. Volunteers have the opportunity to tell Level 4 Disorganized Attachment Story that answers the question, "What does disorganized attachment look like?" Remember to tell these stories using only facial expression, body language, movement or non-

TOXIC RELATIONSHIPS
DISORGANIZED ATTACHMENT AND TRAUMA

verbal interactions with others. Have fun with this! You are "Going Hollywood."

6. Your facilitator will keep track of time for you, and will let you know when it is time to restart the video.

Facilitator Note: Restart the video.

Dismissive, distracted and disorganized attachments are painful.
- Our level of pain is higher than our level of joy.
- This is experienced as trauma and ongoing relational distress.
- But it gets worse!

Non-secure attachments produce ongoing trauma.
- Non-secure attachments lead to a level of pain that exceeds our joy capacity, and this means that we tend to live in ongoing trauma and distress.
- Non-secure attachments continue to make the problem worse because they cause increasing levels of pain and distress – and decrease our levels of joy.
- Our level of trauma worsens.
- We are continually re-traumatized by our non-secure attachments.

Lack of secure attachment diminishes capacity for life and relationships.
- Non-secure attachment hurts relationships throughout my lifespan.

Diminished capacity: trauma

What is trauma?
- Trauma is an experience or series of experiences that overwhelm our emotional capacity to handle the experience. As a result of being overwhelmed, we are diminished as persons, are not able to "act like ourselves" and are unable to live from the heart that Jesus gave us.

The issues with trauma:
- How far did you fall?
- What did you hit?
- How was your landing?

Trauma and suffering
- Trauma is anything that reduces who we are, or who we understand ourselves to be. The unregulated emotional intensity of the traumatic event reduces us to less than we were before.
- Suffering: "Those who suffer are at peace with themselves and the world. Sufferers may find their capacities drastically reduced, even to the point of death, but the continue to be themselves with the capacity and dominion they have left." Thomas Gerlach
- Jesus is our example.

Type A trauma
- The absence of necessary good things.

Type A: the absence of necessary good things:
- Inhibits the development of capacity.
- Abandonment, rejection, malnutrition

YOUR NOTES

TOXIC RELATIONSHIPS
DISORGANIZED ATTACHMENT AND TRAUMA

- Isolation, lack of love
- No encouragement
- Insecure attachments

Type B trauma
- Bad things that happen

Type B: bad things that happen
- Overwhelms existing capacity
- Murder, rape, assault
- Molestation, incest, child abuse
- Humiliation, betrayal, contempt
- "First-person shooter" video games

The loss of the ability to regulate the intensity of feelings is the most far-reaching effect of early trauma and neglect. (van der Kolk)

Medicate to regulate

BEEPS
- BEEPS are attachments to Behaviors, Events, Experiences, People or Substances that are used to regulate emotions, increase pleasure or decrease pain.

BEEPS
- Attachments to BEEPS help us medicate – to artificially regulate – positive and negative emotions as well as pain.

BEEPS
- Attachments to BEEPS take the place of secure attachments to God and significant others.

BEEPS
- There are many different types of BEEPS. Examples can include:
- Behaviors: Work
- Events: Thrill Seeking
- Experiences: Sex
- People: Relationships
- Substances: Alcohol

The BEEPS cycle is relational
- Attachment pain > reduced capacity > BEEPS attachments > damaged relationships > attachment pain.
- That's why recovery must also be relational.

The Twelve Steps are a relational program of recovery.
- Relationship with God
  - Steps 1, 2, 3 and 11.
- Relationship with Self
  - Steps 4, 5, 6, 7 and 10.
- Relationship with Others
  - Steps 8, 9, and 12.
- When these relationships grow in balance, our recovery will also remain balanced.
- Without growth in all 3 of these relationships, recovery will be out of balance, and will not stand.

TOXIC RELATIONSHIPS
DISORGANIZED ATTACHMENT AND TRAUMA

When we apply the Twelve Steps relationally to attachment pain
- Our hearts can heal from trauma.

We can attach to others in joy
- Our recovery is Thriving!

EXERCISE: INTRODUCTION TO THE IMMANUEL PROCESS *30 Minutes*

Facilitator Note: The name "Immanuel" means "God with us," and is one of the names that is used to describe Jesus in the Old and New Testaments. The Immanuel Process is an exercise that is designed to help participants recognize the presence of Jesus in their lives.

Though Jesus has promised to be with us always, (Matt 28:20), we are not always aware that He is present with us. Like the disciples on the Emmaus Road, (Luke 24:13-32) it is possible for Jesus to be with us – but for us to not perceive His presence. The Immanuel Process is based upon the Scriptural truth that Jesus is always with us – and that He can open the eyes of our heart so that we can perceive His presence with us. Our life will forever change as we learn to trust and rely on the comforting presence, joy and ever-present love of the One who is with us.

This exercise introduces The Immanuel Process by asking participants to remember a time or experience in which they felt that Jesus was very near to them. This could be described as a "peak experience" with Jesus, in which they were unusually aware of His presence. As participants remember their encounter with Jesus, they will be asked to describe the event and their feeling during the experience. We will practice this exercise in different formats for several weeks.

Recalling "close encounters of the Jesus kind" helps participants become more aware of how much Jesus wants to be part of their daily life. It helps participants learn to see themselves as He does: as an absolute joy and delight. As they practice this exercise, participants learn that throughout their day, they can learn to ask Jesus, "Where are you now? Will you help me to perceive your presence now?" By remembering times of great joy and peace with Jesus, participants will also build a foundation from which they can later begin to allow Jesus to take them to non-peaceful places in their past.

The Immanuel Process is an important part of trauma recovery. Just as memories of past trauma can affect our lives in the present, memories of joy with Jesus can also powerfully affect our lives today. As we become intentional about recalling our experiences with Jesus, our memories of those moments can lay a new foundation for relational recovery from trauma.

As you lead this exercise, please keep in mind that some participants may not be able to describe a "peak experience" or time in which they felt particularly close with Jesus. This may be due to a variety of factors. Some may have never asked Jesus to be part of their life, and as a result, have had no real awareness of His presence. Others may have experienced severe wounding or trauma, which has made it difficult for them to remember a time in which they felt very close to Jesus. In some cases, participants may have too much fear to engage in this process – or have just never learned to recognize the presence of Jesus.

YOUR NOTES

TOXIC RELATIONSHIPS
DISORGANIZED ATTACHMENT AND TRAUMA

It is important that you explain these possible obstacles before the exercise begins. It is also important that everyone, regardless of personal experience, can participate as active listeners in the small group process that is part of this exercise. Sometimes, listening to another person describe a joyful and meaningful encounter with Jesus can help create a desire for a relationship with Jesus in someone who does not yet know Him. Descriptions of joyful and life giving encounters with Jesus can help reduce fear in those who are fearful, and can also provide useful examples of what the presence of Jesus feels like for those who have never learned to recognize Him. Finally, Jesus knows if someone is just in too much pain from trauma - or the blockages caused by trauma – to easily perceive His presence. It is important to reassure these participants that Jesus will provide other people to help provide what they need to break through these barriers. Everyone, regardless of their ability to perceive the presence of Jesus can benefit from the small group sharing that is part of this exercise. Joy bonds will build as joyful stories about Jesus are shared.

Finally, please keep in mind that a genuine experience or encounter with Jesus will always be consistent with the character and nature of Jesus as revealed in the Scripture.

1. Break into small groups of 3-5 people.

2. Your facilitator will introduce you to the Immanuel Process Exercise. This exercise will help you recognize times in your life in which you felt particularly close with Jesus – or were aware of His presence.
    a. "Immanuel" means "God with us."
    b. Jesus has promised to always be with us – Matt 28:20.
    c. It is possible for Jesus to be with us – and be totally unaware of His presence. It is also possible for Jesus to help us recognize His presence. (Luke 24:13-32).
    d. Recalling our experience of God is scriptural. (John 14:26, Matt 16:9, Psalm 42).
    e. Just as trauma can be a part of our memory – so can the presence of Jesus.

3. Your facilitator will share with you a time when he/she experienced the presence of God in a way that was powerful, meaningful and memorable. He/she will maintain eye contact with you as he/she describes:
    a. What happened in the experience he/she is remembering.
    b. What emotions he/she felt.
    c. What his/her body felt like when he/she was with Jesus.
    d. What he/she did when he/she experienced His presence.
    e. How does it feels to be with Jesus.

4. Your facilitator will ask each of you to close your eyes, and ask Jesus to help you remember a time when you felt very close to Him. As your eyes are closed, your facilitator may help you by quietly asking the questions listed below. You do not need to answer these questions aloud; the questions are only to help you focus on the memory of your experience with Jesus. Your facilitator will help you by keeping track of time during this portion of the exercise, and let you know when it is time to open your eyes.
    a. What is happening in the experience you are remembering?
    b. What emotions are you feeling?
    c. What does your body feel like when you are with Jesus?
    d. What are you doing in that memory?
    e. How does it feel to be with Jesus?

5. Your facilitator will let you know when to open your eyes, and ask for volunteers

TOXIC RELATIONSHIPS
DISORGANIZED ATTACHMENT AND TRAUMA

to begin sharing for 2 minutes about their experience with their small group. Your facilitator will help you keep track of time as you share. Remember to stay relational by making eye contact as you describe:
   a. The experience with Jesus you just remembered.
   b. The emotions you felt in the memory.
   c. What your body felt like.
   d. What you did when you felt the presence of Jesus.
   e. How does it feel to remember this experience with Jesus?

6. When each participant has had the opportunity to share their experience with their small group, your facilitator will ask volunteers to describe what it feels like to experience the presence of Jesus with the entire group. Use one or two words to describe your feelings.

CLOSE THE GROUP WITH PRAYER

need sander

TOXIC RELATIONSHIPS
DISORGANIZED ATTACHMENT AND TRAUMA

QUESTIONS FOR FURTHER DISCUSSION OR FOLLOW-UP

1. How do you define disorganized attachment?

2. What characterizes a relationship between parent and their child in disorganized attachment?

3. What issues in the life of a parent can lead to the development of disorganized attachment?

4. Why do you think that addictions can play a role in the development of a disorganized attachment? Can addictions lead to disorganized attachment?

5. Why do disorganized attachments lead to such toxic relationships?

6. Have you ever been in a relationship with a person who had disorganized attachment? What was that relationship like?

7. Why does "biblical submission" fail as a strategy for dealing with domestic violence?

8. Have you been able to identify your own attachment style? How has this influenced your ability to develop a secure attachment with God?

9. Has your own non-secure attachment style interfered with your ability to have satisfying relationships in life? How have these non-secure attachments affected your attachments with others throughout your life? Be as specific as you can.

10. How do you define trauma? Why is an understanding of capacity so essential for this definition?

11. What is the difference between trauma and suffering? How could Jesus have endured the cross – but still continue to act like himself in the midst of His suffering?

12. What is the difference between Trauma A and Trauma B? Why is it important to understand the difference?

13. How do Trauma A and Trauma B each affect our capacity?

14. Have you experienced Trauma A or Trauma B? How have these influenced your capacity, life and relationships?

15. Why is it so important for recovery to be relational?

16. How can the Twelve Steps help keep our recovery balanced?

17. What did you experience during The Immanuel Process exercise? How did you feel during the exercise?

TOXIC RELATIONSHIPS
DISORGANIZED ATTACHMENT AND TRAUMA

OPTIONAL 12-STEP QUESTIONS

1. Why is the BEEPS cycle relational?

2. Did one or both of your parents use BEEPS? How did this influence your attachments with them? Were their attachments with you disorganized?

3. Have you ever had a truly secure and satisfying relationship – or have your relationships been continually sabotaged by non-secure attachments? Explain.

4. How did you handle the relational pain when relationships did not work – or were unsatisfying? What BEEPS did you use to medicate the pain?

5. Has your use of BEEPS made your attachment pain worse? How?

6. How has your use of BEEPS diminished your capacity for life and relationships?

7. Would you describe your attachment with BEEPS as dismissive, distracted or disorganized? Why?

8. Has your use of BEEPS caused your relationships with others to become increasingly dismissive, distracted or disorganized? Why – or why not?

9. How do you define trauma? How has your use of BEEPS been traumatic to you and others?

10. Have you experienced Trauma A and/or B? List at least 3 ways in which these have affected your life, capacity and relationships.

11. Do you use BEEPS to medicate the pain of Trauma A or Trauma B? How has this diminished your capacity and made your level of pain worse?

12. Why is it so important for your relationships with God, yourself and others to grow in recovery? What happens if these relationships get out of balance?

13. How can the Twelve Steps help your relationships to remain balanced as your recovery grows?

14. What did you experience during the Immanuel Process exercise? How did you feel during the exercise? How were these emotions different from the feelings you get after using BEEPS?

8 TRAUMA, HOPE AND RECOVERY
TRAUMA

OPEN THE GROUP

- Ask for a volunteer to open the group in prayer.

EXERCISE: A MOMENT WITH JESUS *10 Minutes*

Facilitator Note: This is a joy and capacity building exercise that helps prepare participants for this week's lesson. It also helps them get ready for this week's Immanuel Process exercise.

To lead this exercise, you will need to share a moment from the past week in which you experienced the presence of Jesus. As you share your story, remember to stay relational with your group by maintaining eye contact. Describe the moment you had with Jesus, the emotions and body sensations you experienced during the experience, and how you felt afterwards.

When you have finished your story, volunteers will have the opportunity to share their experiences with Jesus in their small groups.

1. Break into small groups of 3-5 people.

2. Your facilitator will ask volunteers to share about a time in the past week when they felt that Jesus was with them. Your facilitator will begin the exercise by sharing a moment from the past week in which he/she was able to perceive the presence of Jesus. Your facilitator will stay relational with you by maintaining eye contact as he/she shares and describes:
   a. The experience he/she had with Jesus.
   b. The emotions he/she felt.
   c. How his/her body felt.
   d. How he/she felt after the experience.

3. Each volunteer can take 2 minutes to share about his/her experience with their small group. Be sure to stay relational by making eye contact as you share your experience with Jesus and describe:
   a. The experience you had with Jesus.
   b. The emotions you felt.
   c. How your body felt.
   d. How you felt after the experience.

4. Your facilitator will help you by keeping track of time.

5. When each group is finished, your facilitator may ask volunteers to share how they feel after the exercise with the entire group. Use one or two words to describe your feelings.

YOUR NOTES

TRAUMA, HOPE AND RECOVERY
TRAUMA

YOUR NOTES

TODAY'S LESSON: Trauma and Recovery

Facilitator Note: Play Session Eight on the Restarting DVD.
- Ask the class to follow along in their workbooks, and take notes as needed.

CLASS NOTES: Trauma and Recovery

Attachment: a quick review:
- Secure
- Dismissive
- Distracted
- Disorganized

Secure attachment:
- Secure attachment results from high joy capacity and synchronized bonds.
- How do non-secure attachments form?

After the Fall:
- Then the eyes of both of them were opened, and they knew that they were naked; and they sewed fig leaves together and made themselves coverings And they heard the sound of the Lord God walking in the garden in the cool of the day, and Adam and his wife hid themselves from the presence of the Lord God among the trees of the garden.
- Then the Lord God called to Adam and said to him, "Where are you?"
- So he said, "I heard Your voice in the garden, and I was afraid because I was naked; and I hid myself."
- And He said, "Who told you that you were naked? Have you eaten from the tree of which I commanded you that you should not eat?"
- Then the man said, "The woman whom You gave to be with me, she gave me of the tree, and I ate."
- And the Lord God said to the woman, "What is this you have done?"
- The woman said, "The serpent deceived me, and I ate." Genesis 3:7-10. NKJV.

Non-secure attachments result from:
- Lack of joy capacity.
- Lack of synchronization.
- Getting stuck in pain without the ability to return to joy.
- These keep us further disconnected from joyful relationships with God and others.

Dismissive attachment: a painful identity
- Avoid relationship
- Low affect
- Negative emotions
- Withdrawal as coping strategy
- Can't synchronize
- Life is safer and feels better alone

Distracted attachment: a painful identity
- Highly needy
- Always trying to attach to receive comfort for distress.
- High affect and drama
- Approach as coping strategy

TRAUMA, HOPE AND RECOVERY
TRAUMA

- Frequent crisis
- Can use "neediness" or distress to manipulate others for attention

Disorganized attachment: a painful identity
- Attachment is source of terror and comfort
- High affect/drama and fearful withdrawal or attack
- Very manipulative
- Hostile/aggressive with peers
- Difficult social relationships
- Abuser or abuse victim

Lack of secure attachment diminishes capacity for life and relationships.
- Non-secure attachment hurts relationships throughout my lifespan.

Diminished capacity: ongoing trauma

What is trauma?
- Trauma is an experience or series of experiences that overwhelm our emotional capacity to handle the experience.
- It also tends to damage other areas of life that are related to the initial trauma.
- As a result of being overwhelmed, we are diminished as persons, are not able to "act like ourselves" and are unable to live from the heart that Jesus gave us.

The issues with trauma:
- How far did you fall?
- What did you hit?
- How was your landing?

Trauma and suffering:
- Trauma is anything that reduced who we are, or who we understand ourselves to be. The unregulated emotional intensity of the traumatic event reduces us to less than we were before it.
- Suffering: "Those who suffer are at peace with themselves and the world. Sufferers may find their capacities drastically reduced, even to the point of death, but they continue to be themselves with the capacities and dominion they have left."
  Thomas Gerlach
- Jesus is our example.

Type A trauma
- The absence of necessary good things.

Type A: the absence of necessary good things
- Inhibits the development of capacity
- Abandonment, rejection, malnutrition
- Isolation, lack of love
- No encouragement
- Insecure attachments

Type B trauma
- Bad things that happen.

Type B: bad things that happen
- Overwhelms existing capacity
- Murder, rape, assault
- Molestation, incest, child abuse

TRAUMA, HOPE AND RECOVERY
TRAUMA

- Humiliation, betrayal, contempt
- "First-person shooter" video games

Trauma A or B can severely impact the control center on multiple levels:
- Level 1: Attachment pain
- Level 2: Pervasive fear
- Level 3: Desynchronized, stuck in negative emotions
- Level 4: Immaturity
- Level 5: Inconsistent identity

Disruption to the control center:
- Degree of pain depends on:
  - Age
  - Severity of trauma
  - Existing capacity
  - Attachments
- It is often sub-cortical.
- May result in unregulated emotions – without the ability to calm yourself.
- Communication between portions of the left and right hemispheres of the brain may temporarily shut down.

Trauma disrupts communication between the left and right hemispheres of the brain.
- Left hemisphere: naming and explaining
- Right hemisphere: knowing and experience
- The first indication of being overwhelmed (as well as the persistent evidence of trauma) is a desynchronization or disconnection between the right and left hemispheres of the brain when what we are experiencing does not fit our explanations about ourselves and our life.
- The right side of the brain takes over until the distress has passed.

Loss of control:
- The prefrontal cortex loses control of the amygdala.

Communication breakdown: right hemisphere
- If things get worse, communication with the PFC breaks down when the capacity and the control center are overwhelmed.
- The amygdala (sub-cortical) runs the control center until the distress/trauma is over.

  When the amygdala is in charge, we visit one of these desks:
  - The Flight Desk:
    - Run and get away.
  - The Fight Desk:
    - Protect ourself and make the distress stop.
  - The Check Out Desk:
    - Shut down until it's over.
  - The Library Desk:
    - Study the problem.

Fear-based thinking dominates.
- The portions of the control center and right brain that are more concerned with primitive impulses of survival often dominate.
- Fear based thinking: Running on adrenaline - terror/rage
  - I can become a non-relational human being
  - I do not think or act like a person

TRAUMA, HOPE AND RECOVERY
TRAUMA

- I cannot distinguish people from objects
- I am not open to logic, reason or persuasion – facts don't work!

Dissociation
- If the trauma and terror/rage persist, I shut down into an energy conservation state known as dissociation.
- "An energy conservation withdrawal state in which all possible brain circuits are shut down after a massive desynchronization. Only the amygdala which can't be shut down is ON, along with the associated regions. This is experienced as "death" at the moment there should have been rest." Dr. Alan Schore.
- It is like dying.

In dissociation:
- We have exhausted our sympathetic arousal of terror and rage.
- A parasympathetic shut down occurs to save energy.

Dissociation is sub-cortical
- It is below our conscious control.

Once dissociation is used to replace rest, the brain will tend to dissociate – rather than learn to rest in the future.
- The dissociative child learns to shut down instead of rest.
- Not learning to rest is bad for us – and for our brain!
- Not learning to rest (serotonin regulation) is the main predictor of mental Illness during the remainder of life.

When the left hemisphere is not communicating with the right hemisphere, our explicit memory is impaired.
- I may no longer remember or be aware that I am present in the trauma, or that it happened to me.

The loss of the ability to regulate the intensity of feelings is the most far-reaching effect of early trauma and neglect. (van der kolk)

Positive feeling traumas and euphoric recall:
- Not all traumas are the result of negative feelings.
- The intensity of positive feelings – or the memory of those feelings - can be traumatic when they overwhelm our capacity to handle those positive feelings.
- This is a critical issue in BEEPS and relapse.

Medicate to regulate

BEEPS
- There are many different types of BEEPS. Examples can include:
- Behaviors: Work
- Events: Thrill Seeking
- Experiences: Sex
- People: Relationships
- Substances: Alcohol

The BEEPS cycle is relational
- Attachment pain> reduced capacity> BEEPS attachments > damaged relationships >attachment pain.
- This cycle of pain must be addressed in recovery.

TRAUMA, HOPE AND RECOVERY
TRAUMA

YOUR NOTES

The Twelve Steps can help us address the pain and trauma of the BEEPS cycle:
- Relationship with God
  - Steps 1, 2, 3 and 11.
- Relationship with self
  - Steps 4, 5, 6, 7 and 10.
- Relationship with others
  - Steps 8, 9, and 12.
- When these relationships grow in balance, our recovery will also remain balanced.
- Without growth in all 3 of these relationships, recovery will be out of balance, and will not stand.
- The 12 Steps can help us address the pain and trauma of the BEEPS cycle only if we are part of a joyful community that can help us heal and grow through our pain.

Thriving builds joyful community to help us heal and grow through the pains of trauma and addiction.
- Unlike many Twelve Step and self-help recovery groups, Thriving specifically identifies Trauma A and Trauma B as significant factors relating to both addiction and relapse.
- Thriving teaches participants the joy and relationship building skills that the brain needs to heal – and remain sober – through the development of secure, healthy attachments with God and others in a mature, life-giving community.

EXERCISE: THE IMMANUEL PROCESS *45 Minutes*

Facilitator Note: We learned last week that the name "Immanuel" means "God with us," and is one of the names that is used to describe Jesus in the Old and New Testaments. The Immanuel Process is an exercise that is designed to help participants recognize the presence of Jesus in their lives.

Though Jesus has promised to be with us always (Matt 28:20), we are not always aware that He is present with us. Like the disciples on the Emmaus Road (Luke 24:13-32,) it is possible for Jesus to be with us – but for us to not perceive His presence. The Immanuel Process is based upon the Scriptural truth that Jesus is always with us – and that He can open the eyes of our heart so that we can perceive His presence with us.

Our life will forever change as we learn to trust and rely on the comforting presence, joy and ever-present love of the One who is with us.

The Immanuel Process can be an important part of trauma recovery. Just as memories of past trauma can affect our lives in the present, memories of joy with Jesus can also powerfully affect our lives today. As we become intentional about recalling our experiences with Jesus, our memories of those moments can lay a new foundation for relational recovery from trauma. These joyful encounters with Jesus can help us build the capacity we need to begin resolving painful life trauma.

Without a level of joy strength that exceeds our level of pain, it is impossible for the brain to remember – or resolve – painful life trauma. Remembering and meditating on joyful moments with Jesus helps build enough capacity so that He is able to lead us into other areas of life that do not feel peaceful. He literally builds enough capacity in us so that we are able to heal by perceiving His presence in difficult areas of life.

TRAUMA, HOPE AND RECOVERY
TRAUMA

One of the most devastating aspects of trauma is that we feel alone, isolated and cut off from others in our pain. When we are able to perceive that Jesus has always been with us – even in the most painful moments of our lives – we discover that we have never been alone. When we experience the presence of Jesus in areas of life that have been painful, we receive comfort, healing and a sense of being deeply connected with Jesus. This experience is at the heart of this week's Immanuel Process exercise.

In last week's the Immanuel Process exercise, participants remembered a time or experience in which they felt that Jesus was very near to them. This was described as a "peak experience" with Jesus, in which they were unusually aware of His presence. As participants reflected on their encounter with Jesus, they learned to describe the event and their feeling during the experience. They were building joy and capacity by experiencing and perceiving the presence of Jesus.

The first part of this week's exercise is identical to last week's Immanuel Process exercise. Participants will again focus on remembering a time or experience with Jesus in which they felt that He was very near to them. As in last week's exercise, they will again be asked to remember the details of the experience, and what their emotions and body felt like when they were with Him. Participants are encouraged to reflect on this experience and to enjoy the presence of Jesus.

After participants have had time to reflect on their experience with Jesus, they will have opportunity to share about their experience in a small group. Sharing about experiences with Jesus builds individual and group capacity, which is important for the second part of this exercise.

In the second part of this week's exercise, participants who have been able to remember a time in which they experienced the presence of Jesus are invited to ask Jesus to show them a place in their life that does not feel peaceful, or in which they did not experience His presence. They will ask Jesus to help them move from their joyful experience with Him into an area of life in which they have not previously felt His presence.

When Jesus shows them a place in which they did not feel His presence, participants will be invited to ask Jesus, "Jesus, where are you now?" and then wait for Him to respond. For those who are having difficulty perceiving Jesus' presence, participants may ask "Jesus, what is keeping me from perceiving your presence now?" and then wait for Him to respond. Participants may also ask "Jesus, is there anything you want me to do now?" and then wait for Him to respond. In this portion of the exercise participants may ask these questions silently, and listen quietly for the answers.

NOTE: If participants do not experience a positive memory with Jesus they should not go on to second part of the exercise but should repeat the first part and look for a positive moment with Jesus instead. If at any point participants feel stuck or distressed, they are encouraged to return to the memory of the peaceful and joyful experience with Jesus that they meditated on in the first part of the exercise. When they feel safe and comfortable enough, they may return again with Jesus to the non-peaceful place.

By moving back and forth as needed between a peaceful experience with Jesus, and one in which they did not perceive His presence, participants avoid feeling overwhelmed and distressed. As the participants are remembering both peaceful and non-peaceful moments – as Jesus leads them – the primary role of the facilitator is to help participants ask questions. At no time should the facilitator suggest or imply anything that participants should feel, perceive, visualize or hear. It is the presence of Jesus, and participant's interactions with Him, that bring healing.

YOUR NOTES

TRAUMA, HOPE AND RECOVERY
TRAUMA

At the conclusion of this part of the exercise, the facilitator will invite all participants to think back to the peaceful and joyful experience with Jesus from the first part of this exercise. The facilitator will invite the group to remember the emotions they felt in His presence. After a few moments of reflection, the facilitator will then ask volunteers to share about their experience in the second part of this exercise with their small group.

It is important that before beginning the second part of this exercise, the facilitator should help participants understand the reasons that some people may have difficulty experiencing the presence of Jesus. These may include:

- Some participants may not be able to describe a "peak experience" or time in which they felt particularly close with Jesus. This may be due to a variety of factors, including the presence of exceptionally severe trauma that has formed blockages that keep them from perceiving His presence. These participants can be encouraged that Jesus often wants to help them by bringing other people into their life that can help them resolve these blockages.
- Some may have never asked Jesus to be part of their life, and as a result, have had no real awareness of His presence. It may be appropriate to ask these participants if they would like to invite Jesus to help them perceive His presence.
- Some participants may experience strong fear that keeps them from perceiving Jesus' presence in non-peaceful areas of life. Because their fear makes it difficult for them to perceive Jesus in distressing areas of life, these participants are encouraged to meditate upon the peaceful experience they meditated on in the first part of the exercise.

For these reasons, it is important that the facilitator invite only those people who have been able to perceive the presence of Jesus in the first part of the exercise to engage in the second part of the exercise. If a participant has been unable to remember a moment in which they were able to experience the presence of Jesus in a way that was meaningful, they are unlikely to have sufficient capacity to experience the presence of Jesus in a non-peaceful moment of life.

Throughout this exercise, it is important for the facilitator to be very sensitive to both the leading of Jesus and to the pain level of the group. Do not rush or hurry through this exercise, and be sure to allow enough time for participants to dialogue with Jesus – and experience His presence. Lead gently, and be sure to allow enough time for all volunteers to share. Please also keep in mind that a genuine experience or encounter with Jesus will always be consistent with the character and nature of Jesus as revealed in the Scripture.

EXERCISE: IMMANUEL PROCESS PART 1

1. Break into small groups of 3-5 people.

2. Your facilitator will introduce you to the Immanuel Process exercise. This exercise will help you recognize times in your life in which you felt particularly close with Jesus – or were aware of His presence. (2-3 Minutes)
   a. "Immanuel" means "God with us."
   b. Jesus has promised to always be with us – Matt 28:20.
   c. It is possible for Jesus to be with us and be totally unaware of His presence. It is also possible for Jesus to help us recognize His presence. (Luke 24:13-32).
   d. Recalling our experience with God is scriptural. (John 14:26, Matt. 16:9, Ps. 42).
   e. Just as trauma can be a part of our memory – so can the presence of Jesus.

TRAUMA, HOPE AND RECOVERY
TRAUMA

YOUR NOTES

3. Your facilitator will share with you a time when he/she experienced the presence of God in a way that was powerful, meaningful and memorable. He/she will maintain eye contact with you as they describe: (2 Minutes)
   a. What happened in the experience he/she is remembering.
   b. What emotions he/she felt.
   c. What his/her body felt like when he/she was with Jesus.
   d. What he/she did when he/she experienced His presence.
   e. How did it feel to be with Jesus?

4. Your facilitator will ask each of you to close your eyes, and ask Jesus to help you remember a time when you felt very close to Him. As your eyes are closed, your facilitator may help you by quietly asking the questions listed below. You do not need to answer these questions aloud; the questions are only to help you focus on the memory of your experience with Jesus. Your facilitator will help you by keeping track of time during this portion of the exercise, and let you know when it is time to open your eyes. (3 Minutes)
   a. What is happening in the experience you are remembering?
   b. What emotions are you feeling?
   c. What does your body feel like when you are with Jesus?
   d. What are you doing in that memory?
   e. How does it feel to be with Jesus?

5. Your facilitator will let you know when to open your eyes, and ask for volunteers to begin sharing for 2 minutes about their experience with their small group. Your facilitator will help you keep track of time as you share. Remember to stay relational by making eye contact as you describe: (10 Minutes)
   a. The experience with Jesus you just remembered.
   b. The emotions you felt in the memory.
   c. What your body felt like.
   d. What you did when you felt the presence of Jesus.
   e. How does it feel to remember this experience with Jesus?

6. When each participant has had the opportunity to share their experience with their small group, your facilitator will ask volunteers to describe what it feels like to experience the presence of Jesus with the entire group. Use one or two words to describe your feelings. (1-2 Minutes)

EXERCISE: IMMANUEL PROCESS PART 2

1. Remain in your small groups of 3-5 people.

2. Your facilitator will introduce the second part of this exercise that involves learning to move from a peaceful place with Jesus in which you can perceive His presence into areas of life that do not feel peaceful or in which you haven't been able to perceive that He is with you. DO NOT TRY THIS SECOND PART IF YOU DID NOT EXPERIENCE JESUS PRESENCE IN THE FIRST PART OF THIS EXERCISE. (5-10 Minutes)

3. Your facilitator will also let you know that if at any point you feel stuck or distressed, you can return to the memory of the joyful and peaceful memory of the experience with Jesus that you described in the first part of the exercise.

4. Your facilitator will also explain the reasons that some people may have difficulty experiencing the presence of Jesus in painful areas of life. These include:
   a. Some participants may not be able to describe a "peak experience" or time in

TRAUMA, HOPE AND RECOVERY
TRAUMA

which they felt particularly close with Jesus. This may be due to a variety of factors, including the presence of exceptionally severe trauma that has formed blockages that keep them from perceiving His presence. These participants can be encouraged that Jesus often wants to help them by bringing other people into their life that can help them resolve these blockages.

  b. Some may have never asked Jesus to be part of their life, and as a result, have had no real awareness of His presence. It may be appropriate to ask these participants if they would like to invite Jesus to help them perceive His presence.
  c. Some participants may experience strong fear that keeps them from perceiving Jesus' presence in non-peaceful areas of life. Because their fear makes it difficult for them to perceive Jesus in distressing areas of life, these participants are encouraged to meditate upon the peaceful experience they meditated on in the first part of the exercise.

5. Your facilitator will ask each of you to close your eyes, and think again about the time you felt very close to Jesus. Your facilitator will help you by quietly asking the questions listed below. Participants who were able to perceive the presence of Jesus in the first part of this exercise are invited to ask Him these questions. You do not need to answer these questions aloud; these are questions for you to ask Jesus. As you ask these questions, be sensitive to His presence and leading. After each question, wait for Jesus to help you. These questions are: (5 Minutes)
   a. Jesus, is there a non-peaceful place in my life that you want to show me?
   b. Where are you in this place? Will you help me to perceive your presence here?
   c. Jesus, what is keeping me from perceiving your presence here?
   d. Jesus, is there anything you want me to do now?
   e. If you did not find a peaceful memory with Jesus in the first part of this Immanuel Process exercise continue looking for a peaceful place with God rather than asking about the non-peaceful places in your life.

6. During this portion of the exercise, your facilitator may help you by reminding you that you can return to the joyful and peaceful memory of your experience with Jesus that you described in the first part of this exercise.

7. At the conclusion of this exercise, your facilitator will invite you to return to the peaceful and joyful memory that you described in the first part of this exercise.

8. Your facilitator will let you know when to open your eyes, and ask for volunteers to begin sharing for 2 minutes in their small group about their experience. Your facilitator will help you keep track of time as you share. Remember to stay relational by making eye contact as you describe: (10 Minutes)
   a. The experience with Jesus you just remembered.
   b. The emotions you felt in the memory.
   c. What your body felt like.
   d. What you did when you felt the presence of Jesus.
   e. How does it feel to remember this experience with Jesus?

9. When everyone has had the opportunity to share in their small group, your facilitator may ask volunteers to share one or two words with the entire group to describe their experience with Jesus in the second part of the exercise. (2 Minutes).

CLOSE THE GROUP WITH PRAYER

TRAUMA, HOPE AND RECOVERY
TRAUMA

QUESTIONS FOR FURTHER DISCUSSION OR FOLLOW-UP

1. Why is a painful identity a problem that is common to dismissive, distracted and disorganized attachments?

2. What happens to the development of capacity with Trauma A? What happens to existing capacity with Trauma B?

3. What do you think happens to our capacity when we experience both Trauma A and Trauma B?

4. What effect does trauma have on each level of the control center?

5. How does trauma influence our ability to self-regulate emotions?

6. Why do you think it is important that many of trauma's impacts on us are sub-cortical?

7. What happens to communication between the left and right hemispheres of the brain when we experience trauma?

8. Being so upset that we "can't think straight" can describe the type of distress we experience when communication breaks down between the left and right hemispheres of the brain. Have you ever had this experience? Describe your experience. What did you do when you were this upset? From what you now know about recovery and the brain, how would you have liked to be able to handle the experience?

9. What can happen to communication between the right pre-frontal cortex and the amygdala if our level of distress is too overwhelming?

10. What are the four things that we can do when we are overwhelmed and the amygdala is in charge?

11. Have you ever been so upset that your only thought was to run away or fight? Describe your experience. What did you do when you were this upset? From what you know about recovery and the brain, how would you have liked to be able to handle the experience?

12. What happens when fear-based thinking dominates us?

13. In your own words, how would you describe dissociation? Why does it happen?

14. Why can positive feelings or euphoric recall be traumatic for the brain?

15. How can Thriving help you heal and grow through the pain of Trauma A and Trauma B?

16. What did you experience during this week's Immanuel Process exercise?

TRAUMA, HOPE AND RECOVERY
TRAUMA

OPTIONAL 12-STEP QUESTIONS

1. Why is recovery from trauma so essential for recovery from BEEPS?

2. How can the Twelve Steps help you to recover from the pain of trauma and attachments to BEEPS?

3. How can dismissive, distracted and disorganized attachment keep you stuck in attachment pain and the BEEPS cycle? Explain.

4. How is the heart that Jesus gave you different from the painful identity that has kept you stuck in trauma and attachments to BEEPS?

5. How have Trauma A and/or Trauma B kept you stuck in cycles of pain that influence your attachments to BEEPS?

6. When we are overwhelmed, communication between the left and right hemispheres of the brain is disrupted. How can this lead to relapse?

7. In recovery, many of us have developed good left-brained relapse prevention plans and thought a lot about how we could avoid using BEEPS. We developed strategies like making phone calls, praying or going to meetings so that we'd know what to do if we felt like using BEEPS. Then, we got so stressed or upset that we used BEEPS anyway, and barely even thought about the plan until later. Has this ever happened to you? Describe this situation. How might this have been different if you had more capacity?

8. Feeling anxious is usually an indication that we are afraid. How do you handle anxiety? What happens to you when your anxiety grows? Have you ever used BEEPS to medicate anxiety? Describe.

9. How do you handle feelings of anger or rage? What happens to you when anger and resentments build? Have you ever used BEEPS as a result? Describe.

10. Can avoiding anxiety and anger work as an effective relapse strategy? From what you have learned in Restarting, what do you need to learn to handle emotions like fear and anger? Where can you find these resources?

11. Have you ever felt like you "just checked out" before you used BEEPS? Describe this experience. What were you feeling before you "checked out?"

12. Why do you think that relapse prevention strategies that focus primarily on the left-brain tend to fail? Why does right-brain training and the development of capacity need to be a part of your recovery?

13. What is euphoric recall? How has euphoric recall been a part of your attachment to BEEPS? What do you need to overcome euphoric recall?

14. How can intense positive emotions contribute to relapse? Has this ever happened to you? Explain.

15. Why do you need a joyful and healing community to recover from the pain of trauma and attachments to BEEPS?

16. What did you experience during this week's Immanuel Process exercise? Do you think that the Immanuel Process can be a helpful part of your recovery program?

9 LEAVING CODEPENDENCY BEHIND
BEEPS MEDICATE TO REGULATE PART 1: SECURE ATTACHMENTS, IDENTITY AND INTERDEPENDENCE

OPEN THE GROUP

- Ask for a volunteer to open the group in prayer.

EXERCISE: A MOMENT WITH JESUS *5 Minutes*

Facilitator Note: This joy and capacity building exercise reviews last week's Immanuel Process exercise. It also reminds participants that they can learn to experience the presence of Jesus throughout the week.

It is helpful for you to begin the exercise by sharing a moment in the past week in which you experienced the presence of Jesus. Please take 1 minute to share your experience – and the emotions you felt – with the group. When you have finished, you may ask volunteers to share for a minute about a moment from the past week in which they experienced the presence of Jesus.

1. Everyone can remain together in a large group for this exercise.

2. Your facilitator will share for one minute about a moment in the past week when he/she experienced the presence of Jesus. Your facilitator will describe that moment and what emotions he/she felt when he/she realized that Jesus was with him/her.

3. Your facilitator will ask volunteers to share about a moment in the past week when they experienced the presence of Jesus.

4. Volunteers each have one minute to share about that moment, and describe the experience and emotions they felt when they realized that Jesus was with them.

5. Your facilitator will help you by keeping track of time.

TODAY'S LESSON: BEEPS Medicate to Regulate Part 1:
Secure Attachments, Identity and Interdependence

Facilitator Note: Play Session Nine on the Restarting DVD.
- Ask the class to follow along in their workbooks, and take notes as needed.

CLASS NOTES: Secure Attachments, Identity and Interdependence.

BEEPS
- BEEPS are attachments to Behaviors, Events, Experiences, People or Substances that are used to regulate emotions, increase pleasure or decrease pain.
- Attachments to BEEPS help us medicate – to artificially regulate – positive and nega-

LEAVING CODEPENDENCY BEHIND
BEEPS MEDICATE TO REGULATE PART 1: SECURE ATTACHMENTS, IDENTITY AND INTERDEPENDENCE

tive emotions as well as pain.
- Attachments to BEEPS take the place of secure attachments to God and significant others.

Attachment can lead to:
- Healthy interdependence or
- Harmful dependency.

Thriving is unique:
- The same mechanism that causes us to attach to BEEPS is the same mechanism that helps us securely attach in joyful relationships with God and others.
- Thriving deals with more than negative attachments and the drive to "medicate to regulate."
- Thriving teaches us to give our brain what it really wants and really craves, and that is joy – and joyful relationships with others.
- Joy means relationship.

How do we build a strong, joyful identity, healthy attachments and interdependent relationships?

We are created for secure attachments with God and others.
- Everything about us is created to be relational.

Adam and Eve were created for secure attachment and healthy interdependence.
- Let us make man in our own image, in our likeness…So God created man in his own image, in the image of God he created him; male and female he created them.
  Genesis 1:26, 27, NKJV
- It is not good for the man to be alone. I will make a helper suitable for him…and He brought her to the man. The man said, "This is now flesh of my flesh…For this reason, a man will leave his father and mother and be united to his wife and they will become one flesh." Genesis 2:18, 22, 23, NKJV

Rhythms of joy and quiet together create secure attachment and identity that is joyful, secure and strong.

High joy capacity helps build a strong identity.
- Increasing capacity helps develop an identity that is strong – even when facing distress.

When others are glad to be with me when I am distressed:
- I can learn to return to joy from negative emotions.
- My attachments and bonds remain secure.
- I can act like myself, even when I'm upset.
- These allow secure attachments to grow, even when I'm distressed or upset.
- My individual and group identities are also strengthened.

Secure attachments with a strong, joyful individual and group identity build healthy interdependence.
- Two are better than one, because they have a good return for their work. If one falls down, his friend can help him up. But pity the man who falls and has no one to help him up! Also, if two lie down together they will keep warm. But how can one keep warm alone? Though one may be overpowered, two can defend themselves. A cord of three strands is not easily broken. Ecc. 4: 10-12, NIV.

LEAVING CODEPENDENCY BEHIND
BEEPS MEDICATE TO REGULATE PART 1: SECURE ATTACHMENTS, IDENTITY AND INTERDEPENDENCE

What do healthy attachments and interdependence look like?

Attachment strength: the strength of attachments to BEEPS are reflected by:
- Intensity:
  - How strongly the BEEPS changes emotions, pleasure and/or pain.
- Intimacy:
  - How strongly we relate to and rely on BEEPS to medicate emotions, pain and pleasure.
- Exclusivity:
  - The degree to which we focus our time, effort and energy on BEEPS – to the exclusion of other people, things or God.

Healthy attachment strength
- Intensity
  - Attachment center functioning -secure attachment
  - Joyful capacity
  - Value systems
  - Control center well regulated
- Intimacy
  - Growing attachment and synchronization
  - Continue to regulate emotions well
  - Joy builds
  - Anticipate joy at reunion
  - Acquired value
- Exclusivity
  - Growing attachment and synchronization
  - Bond together for life
  - Give and receive life appropriately
  - Maintain other important relationships
- Interdependence
  - Increased maturity and capacity
  - Increased synchronization, mutual mind
  - Open to receive from others – but bonded relationship is primary
  - Family forms

Healthy interdependence: married and singles:
- Both married and singles can form strong bonds that are intense, intimate, and exclusive – and lead to healthy interdependence.
- Both married and singles can form bonds for life that are intense, intimate and exclusive with parents, siblings, extended family, spiritual family and friends.
- The primary differences are the degree of exclusivity and sexual nature of the bonds between married couples.

Intensity
- Something about the other person gets your attention.
- Something says "pay attention to him/her."
- Something feels good about being with them.
- It is fun!

Intimacy
- As the relationship grows, you spend more time together.
- You share friends and friendships together
- It is fun to be together
- The relationship grows increasingly close.

LEAVING CODEPENDENCY BEHIND
BEEPS MEDICATE TO REGULATE PART 1: SECURE ATTACHMENTS, IDENTITY AND INTERDEPENDENCE

Intimacy
- Your attachment center lights up when you are with them or think about them.
- You are able to regulate emotions, pleasure and pain independently, but are synchronizing with the other person.
- Love grows until you know that you want to spend the rest of your life in relationship with them.

Exclusivity
- The relationship reaches a level in which your bond is exclusive.
- The relationship you have with your bonded partner, parent, child, sibling, spouse or friend is reserved for only one person – them!
- When your attachment is exclusive and healthy, interdependence helps your bonds grow and mature.

A secure, joyful identity leads to secure and interdependent adult attachments.

What does healthy interdependence feel like? What does healthy interdependence look like?
- Pause for a Level 4+ Healthy Interdependence Story
- Pause for a Level 4 Healthy Interdependence Story

EXERCISE: TELLING LEVEL 4+ AND LEVEL 4 HEALTHY INTERDEPENDENCE STORIES *35 Minutes*

Facilitator Note: The purpose of these exercises is to help participants apply the concepts they have learned about healthy interdependence by telling Level 4+ and Level 4 stories. The exercises help build joyful capacity, strengthen group bonds, and make it easier for participants to recognize healthy interdependence by helping them discover what these relationships feel like and look like.

In the first part of the exercise, participants will have the opportunity to tell Level 4+ stories about healthy interdependence. As you recall from previous lessons, Level 4+ stories combine elements of both the left hemisphere (words) and right hemisphere (emotions) of the brain to describe an experience. Since you will be telling a Level 4+ story about secure healthy interdependence, be sure to complete your "Preparing My 4 + Healthy Interdependence Story Worksheet" and practice telling your story ahead of time. It is also a good idea to review the instructions for telling Level 4+ stories from Week 4.

In the second part of the exercise, participants will have the opportunity to tell Level 4 stories about healthy interdependence. Level 4 stories are non-verbal stories, in which participants act out the story they are describing using facial expression, body language, and movement. This exercise allows the right hemisphere of the brain to express itself – without using words. Level 4 stories are a lot of fun for groups. It may help to describe Level 4 stories as an opportunity to "Go to Hollywood," because it gives everyone a chance to try out their acting skills. Because you will be telling a Level 4 story about healthy interdependence, be sure to prepare your story in advance.

Part 1: Preparing to tell a Level 4+ Healthy Interdependence Story
To help participants prepare to tell their Level 4+ Healthy Interdependence Story, it is helpful to do several things. First, make sure participants locate their "Preparing My Level 4+ Healthy Interdependence Story Worksheet" in their workbook. Briefly review

LEAVING CODEPENDENCY BEHIND
BEEPS MEDICATE TO REGULATE PART 1: SECURE ATTACHMENTS, IDENTITY AND INTERDEPENDENCE

each characteristic of a Level 4+ story listed on the worksheet with them.

Second, it is important to help those who have never experienced a relationship that is characterized by healthy interdependence know how to complete their worksheet and tell a Level 4+ story. While participants who have experienced healthy interdependence can complete their worksheet and describe a situation based on their experience, those who have never experienced healthy interdependence have two options. First, they could describe a situation in which they observed a healthy interdependent relationship between others. They can complete their worksheet and tell a Level 4+ story based on that experience. Second, they could complete their worksheet based on what they believe a relationship with healthy interdependence might feel like and look like. They can describe the emotions, body sensations and what it would be like to "act like themselves" in such a relationship.

Please be aware that some participants may have never experienced or seen a relationship between two people that is characterized by healthy interdependence. However, they may report to you that their relationship with God is characterized by healthy interdependence. In this case, please ask them to complete their worksheet based on what they think a relationship with another person would be like – if it shared the same characteristics as the healthy interdependent relationship they describe with God.

Third, tell your own Level 4+ story about healthy interdependence. The best way for participants to learn to tell a Level 4+ story about healthy interdependence is to hear one. When you have finished your story, follow the procedures we have learned previously, and allow your group to give you feedback about your story. The purpose of feedback in Level 4+ stories is to help the storyteller determine if the story met all the guidelines for a Level 4+ story listed on the worksheet. Read each characteristic on the worksheet, and ask your group if your story met each one.

When feedback is complete, it is time for participants to take 5 minutes and complete their own Level 4+ Healthy Interdependence Story Worksheet. When they are finished, volunteers may begin sharing their stories with their small group. Volunteers will have 3 minutes to share their story, followed by 2 minutes of group feedback.

Before the groups begin sharing, it is a good idea to ask participants to raise their hands if they get stuck, have questions or need help once small group sharing begins. Be ready to help as needed.

Part 2: Preparing to tell a Level 4 Healthy Interdependence Story
In the second part of the exercise, volunteers will have the opportunity to "Go Hollywood" and share Level 4 stories about healthy interdependence with the entire group. These stories can illustrate the experience described on the Level 4+ worksheets – or they can also be impromptu depictions of healthy interdependence. Have fun with these stories!

To prepare your group for this exercise, briefly review with them the characteristics of a Level 4 story. Next, tell a Level 4 story about healthy interdependence. This is the best way for them to learn this exercise. After you tell your story, you may ask for volunteers to tell their own Level 4 story about healthy interdependence.

Exercise Part 1: Level 4+ Stories About Healthy Interdependence *(30 Minutes)*

1. Break into small groups of 3 people.

2. Please locate your "Preparing My 4 + Healthy Interdependence Story Worksheet"

LEAVING CODEPENDENCY BEHIND
BEEPS MEDICATE TO REGULATE PART 1: SECURE ATTACHMENTS, IDENTITY AND INTERDEPENDENCE

in your workbook. In the first part of this exercise, you will tell a story about a relationship you have had that is characterized by healthy interdependence. Your facilitator will review the characteristics of a Level 4+ story with you. (5 Minutes).

   a. Please make sure that your story is not so emotionally intense that it overwhelms others.
   b. It helps if this is a story that you have told before – this makes it easier to share.
   c. It is a good idea to avoid stories that may cause you or others feelings of shame or embarrassment.
   d. Make sure that the story is about your feelings and that you are involved in the story.
   e. Be sure that your story clearly illustrates a specific feeling.
   f. As you tell your story, let your face and voice reflect the emotion you are describing.
   g. As you maintain eye contact with others in your small group, it will help you stay connected relationally with them.
   h. Write a brief description of the situation you want to share. You only need to write down enough details to help you remember the story – and be able to share it.
   i. Write the feeling words that describe the emotions that you felt during the story. It helps to list each one.
   j. Write down how your body felt during the situation you are describing. It may be things like "My stomach was in a knot" or "My shoulders felt tight" or "My muscles felt relaxed."
   k. Describe what you did in the story that illustrates how you like to act in a healthy interdependent relationship.

3. Your facilitator will explain how to complete your "Preparing My 4 + Healthy Interdependence Story Worksheet."
   a. If you have experienced a healthy interdependent relationship, complete your worksheet by describing an event from your relationship.
   b. If you have never experienced healthy interdependence, you may describe a healthy interdependent relationship that you have seen between others. Complete your worksheet by describing a time in which you observed this relationship.
   c. If you have never seen or experienced a healthy interdependent relationship, you may complete your worksheet and describe what you think this kind of relationship might be like. What emotions do you think you'd feel, what might your body feel like, and how do you think you would act in a healthy interdependent relationship?

4. Your facilitator will tell a 3 minute Level 4+ Healthy Interdependence Story, followed by 2 minutes of feedback. To help you during the feedback session, your facilitator will read each element of a 4+ story listed on the worksheet, and ask you if the story contained each element. Remember that feedback:
   a. Is based on helping a storyteller determine if their story contained all the elements of a 4+ story listed on the worksheet.
   b. Is not based on criticism or advice about the experience or feelings described.

5. Take 5 minutes to complete your Level 4+ story worksheet. Your facilitator will assist you by keeping track of time, and will let you know when volunteers may begin sharing their stories with their small group.

6. Your facilitator will ask for volunteers in each small group to begin telling their story. You will have 3 minutes to tell your story and your facilitator will keep track

LEAVING CODEPENDENCY BEHIND
BEEPS MEDICATE TO REGULATE PART 1: SECURE ATTACHMENTS, IDENTITY AND INTERDEPENDENCE

of time for you. If at any point your group is stuck or has a question, please raise your hand, and your facilitator will come help you.

7. After the first joy story, each group can take 2 minutes to give feedback on the story. Use the "Preparing My 4 + Healthy Interdependence Story Worksheet" as a guideline to help the storyteller discover if they were able to share all the elements of a 4+ story listed on the worksheet. Be encouraging and positive! Your facilitator will keep track of time for you, and let you know when it is time for the next person to share their story.

8. Your facilitator will let you know when it is time for a second person in each small group to begin their 3-minute Level 4+ Healthy Interdependence Story, followed by 2 minutes of feedback. Your facilitator will keep track of time for you and let you know when it is time for the next person to share their story.

9. Your facilitator will let you know when it is time for the third person in each small group to begin their 3-minute Level 4+ Healthy Interdependence Story, followed by 2 minutes of feedback. Your facilitator will keep track of time for you.

Exercise Part 2: Level 4 Stories About Healthy Interdependence *(5 Minutes)*

1. You may remain in your small groups as your facilitator reviews the characteristics of Level 4 stories with you.
    a. Level 4 stories are non-verbal stories told without using words.
    b. Level 4 stories rely on the right hemisphere of the brain to describe a feeling, experience, sensation, event or story.
    c. In Level 4 stories, participants act out the story and emotions they are describing using only facial expression, body language, movement or non-verbal interactions with others.

2. Your facilitator will tell a Level 4 Healthy Interdependence Story for the entire group that illustrates what healthy interdependence looks like.

3. Volunteers have the opportunity to tell Level 4 Healthy Interdependence Stories to the entire group.
    a. Remember to tell these stories using only facial expression, body language, movement or non-verbal interactions with others.
    b. Your Level 4 stories can illustrate the experience you described on your Level 4+ worksheet, or they can be spontaneous depictions of healthy interdependence.
    c. Have fun with this! You are "Going to Hollywood."

4. Your facilitator will keep track of time for you, and will let you know when it is time to restart the video.

Facilitator Note: Restart the video.

What happens to my identity and attachments when my capacity for joy is low and I can't effectively regulate negative emotions?

Life is pain-centered, and this makes relationships and attachment difficult.
- When my level of pain exceeds my level of joy, I experience trauma.
- I get stuck in ongoing relational distress and further trauma.
- My attachments and identity are centered in ongoing pain.

YOUR NOTES

LEAVING CODEPENDENCY BEHIND
BEEPS MEDICATE TO REGULATE PART 1: SECURE ATTACHMENTS, IDENTITY AND INTERDEPENDENCE

When relationships are painful and my personal and group identity is weak, I can't get back to joy and get stuck in:
- Level 1: Attachment pain
- Level 2: Life is bad and scary
- Level 3: Negative emotions
- Level 4: Immaturity
- Level 4+: Inconsistent identity

I will experience ongoing pain and "Medicate to Regulate."

BEEPS
- Attachments to Behaviors, Events, Experiences, People and Substances that are used to regulate emotions, increase pleasure or decrease pain.

BEEPS
- There are many different types of BEEPS. Examples can include:
- Behaviors: Work
- Events: Thrill Seeking
- Experiences: Sex
- People: Relationships
- Substances: Alcohol

BEEPS and Steps 6 and 7
- Step 6: Were entirely ready to have God remove all these defects of character.
- Step 7: Humbly asked Him to remove our shortcomings.

Steps 6 and 7 teach us:
- Life, relationships and recovery thrive when we stop relying on our own limited abilities to change ourselves – but on God who has no limits.
- We cannot change our lives, brains or BEEPS apart from humility and relationship with God
- Change requires the loving involvement of God and others empowered by joy!

My relationships with others can become empowered by joy
- I can be free from attachments to BEEPS
- I can attach to God and to others in joy!

EXERCISE: MAGGIE'S STORY *5 Minutes*

Facilitator Note: The purpose of this exercise is to allow participants to respond to Maggie's story in this week's video. In this exercise, volunteers will have the opportunity to use one or two words to describe their feelings after watching Maggie's story.

To facilitate this exercise, please review the video prior to group.

1. You can remain in your seats and do not need to break into small groups for this exercise. The purpose of this exercise is to help you describe your feelings after listening to Maggie's story in this week's video.

2. Your facilitator will ask volunteers to share how they feel after watching Maggie's story. Use one or two words to describe your feelings.

LEAVING CODEPENDENCY BEHIND
BEEPS MEDICATE TO REGULATE PART 1: SECURE ATTACHMENTS, IDENTITY AND INTERDEPENDENCE

CLOSE THE GROUP WITH PRAYER

OPTIONAL EXERCISE: PART 1 - DON'T TALK *20 Minutes*

Facilitator Note: The goal of this exercise is to help participants apply what they have learned about healthy interdependence to relationships in which BEEPS are involved. In this exercise, you will use a song describing a conversation between a woman and a man who is drinking too much.

For this exercise, you will need a copy of the song "Don't Talk" by Dennis Drew and Natalie Merchant recorded by 10,000 Maniacs. This song is available on their CDs "In My Tribe" or "10,000 Maniacs MTV Unplugged." Due to copyright and licensing restrictions, we cannot provide you with a copy of the song.

You can purchase these CDs through online vendors or stores where CDs are sold. The song "Don't Talk" may also be purchased and downloaded separately through online music vendors.

If you do not wish to play the song, you may read participants the words to the song. If you choose to play the song, make sure that you have the appropriate music player and speakers available for your group.

Be sure that you preview this song before you lead this exercise.

1. Break into small groups of 3-5 people.

2. In this exercise, you will be using the song "Don't Talk," which describes a conversation between a woman and a man who is drinking too much. The goal of this exercise is to help you apply what you've learned about healthy interdependence to relationships in which BEEPS are involved.

3. Your facilitator may play this song for you – or may read the song lyrics to you.

4. As you listen to the song, pay attention to:
   a. The relationship between the woman and the man.
   b. The impact BEEPS are having on the man who is drinking too much.
   c. The impact of BEEPS upon the woman.

5. When the song is finished, you will have 10 minutes to share the answers to these questions with your group:
   a. What kind of impact are BEEPS having on the man and woman in the song?
   b. What is the difference between their relationship and healthy interdependence?
   c. How are BEEPS keeping them from developing healthy interdependence?

6. Your facilitator will help you by keeping track of time.

7. After 10 minutes of sharing, you may remain in your groups, and your facilitator will lead you in a short relaxation exercise.

YOUR NOTES

LEAVING CODEPENDENCY BEHIND
BEEPS MEDICATE TO REGULATE PART 1: SECURE ATTACHMENTS, IDENTITY AND INTERDEPENDENCE

OPTIONAL EXERCISE: PART 2 - LEARNING TO BREATHE DEEPLY
2 Minutes

1. Follow your facilitator's instructions as you do this exercise.

2. Remain in your small groups. Stand up, and make sure that you have 3-4 feet of clear space around you.

3. Imagine that you are a marionette – a puppet – with a string running from the base of your spine to the top of your head. Imagine that the string is gently pulled upwards and your back, neck and head are perfectly aligned. Your head is at rest and comfortably settled in line with your back and spine. You are looking forward, and your head is settled in comfortably.

4. Bend your knees slightly. You are standing still in a comfortable position.

5. Place your hand over your stomach.

6. Take such a deep breath that you feel your stomach expand as you breathe. Follow your facilitator's instructions as you breathe deeply for a few moments.

7. Your facilitator will keep track of time for you as you relax and breathe deeply.

CLOSE THE GROUP WITH PRAYER

LEAVING CODEPENDENCY BEHIND
BEEPS MEDICATE TO REGULATE PART 1: SECURE ATTACHMENTS, IDENTITY AND INTERDEPENDENCE

QUESTIONS FOR FURTHER DISCUSSION OR FOLLOW-UP

1. Why is it important for you to know that you are designed for secure attachments and healthy interdependence?

2. What do you need to begin to build an identity that is joyful, secure and strong?

3. We often try to avoid, deny or minimize negative emotions in the mistaken belief that these will always damage or destroy our attachments to others. What really happens to your attachments with others when you try to deny, avoid or minimize negative emotions in your relationship with them? Do our attachments become more – or less secure?

4. What happens to our individual identity and attachments with others when they are glad to be with us when we are experiencing a negative emotion?

5. Why do we need a strong, joyful individual identity to build a healthy group identity?

6. How do you define intensity, intimacy and exclusivity?

7. How can intensity, intimacy and exclusivity describe the strength of your attachments?

8. Have you ever tried to form an attachment with someone – when it didn't feel good to be with them? How did this affect your attachment with them?

9. Why are intensity – and a healthy control center – so important for the development of intimacy in healthy attachments? What happens to intensity if my control center does not function well?

10. How can exclusivity be a healthy part of secure attachment?

11. What characterizes healthy interdependency in relationships? How would you describe it?

12. Can both single and married people develop healthy interdependence in relationships? Why? What is the primary difference between healthy interdependence in the bonds shared in a marriage, and the bonds shared by others?

13. Have you ever been in a relationship with healthy interdependence? Describe your relationship. What was it like? How did it feel? If you have never been in a relationship like this, what do you think it would feel like – and look like?

14. What happens to our identity if our capacity for joy is low, and we tend to get stuck in negative emotions? How does this affect our attachments, and ability to form strong and secure group bonds?

15. Why is it so easy to develop an attachment to BEEPS when our individual and group identity is weak?

16. What do you need to develop a stronger individual group and individual identity? Where are the resources you need?

LEAVING CODEPENDENCY BEHIND
BEEPS MEDICATE TO REGULATE PART 1: SECURE ATTACHMENTS, IDENTITY AND INTERDEPENDENCE

OPTIONAL 12-STEP QUESTIONS

1. In your own words, how would you describe Steps 6 & 7?

2. According to these steps, God is a vital part of our recovery. Why is it so important for God to be involved in helping you overcome your character defects and shortcomings?

3. Do you have character defects that you would like to have God remove? Describe these character defects. How do they affect your life and recovery? Are you entirely ready for Him to remove them?

4. Have you ever asked God to remove a character defect from your life – but then been unwilling to let go of it? What happened? Describe your experience.

5. Are there character defects you are not entirely ready to have God remove? Why are you holding on to them? What do you need to release them?

6. How do you define healthy interdependence? How have your attachments to BEEPS interfered with your ability to form healthy interdependence with others?

7. Have you ever experienced healthy interdependence in a relationship? Describe this relationship. What was it like? How did it feel? If you have never been in a relationship like this, what do you think it would feel like – and look like?

8. How do you answer the question, "Who am I?" How do you describe yourself?

9. Do you think that most of your relationships are rooted in joy – or pain? Why?

10. Who are the people that you like to spend time with the most? Do these relationships help make your identity and bonds stronger – or weaker? Explain.

11. What does the word "shortcomings" mean to you? Can "shortcomings" include things like weak attachments, not knowing how to develop healthy relationships and a painful personal and group identity?

12. What are the shortcomings that you would most like God to remove from you? How do you "humbly" ask God to remove your shortcomings? Write down what you would say.

13. What do you think will happen if you humbly ask God to remove your shortcomings? How long will it take Him to remove them?

14. Asking God to remove your shortcomings also means that you would like God to fill you with new and good things. What gifts would you like to receive from God to replace your shortcomings? Be specific!

15. Would you like to ask God to remove your shortcomings? Explain.

10 ATTACHMENTS THAT KILL: HOW ADDICTIONS REWIRE YOUR BRAIN
BEEPS ATTACHMENT AND IDENTITY - MEDICATE TO REGULATE PART 2: HARMFUL DEPENDENCY

OPEN THE GROUP

- Ask for a volunteer to open the group in prayer.

EXERCISE: APPRECIATION AND HEALTHY INTERDEPENDENCE *10 Minutes*

Facilitator Note: In this appreciation exercise, volunteers have the opportunity to share about an experience they had with God or another person in the past week for which they are grateful. Volunteers also have the option of sharing gratitude for a moment in the past week in which they experienced healthy interdependence in their relationship with God or another person. This exercise helps build individual and group capacity, which are particularly important in light of the discussion of attachments to BEEPS that are the focus of this week's lesson.

To lead this exercise, you will need to share your own appreciation moment with the group. Be sure to describe the experience for which you are grateful, along with the emotions and body sensations you felt. Remember to stay relational as you share.

Volunteers can then begin their stories.

1. Break into small groups of 3 people.

2. Your facilitator will ask you to think about a moment from the past week in which you had either:
   a. An experience with God or another person for which you are grateful.
   b. An experience of healthy interdependence in your relationship with God or another person for which you are grateful.

3. Your facilitator will share his/her own appreciation moment from the past week with the entire group. While sharing, your facilitator will:
   a. Maintain eye contact.
   b. Identify the experience for which he/she is grateful.
   c. Describe the emotions he/she felt during the experience.
   d. Describe what his/her body felt like during the experience.

4. Your facilitator will ask volunteers to take turns sharing about their own experience with their small group. Each volunteer will have 2 minutes to share. Remember to:
   a. Maintain eye contact while sharing.
   b. Identify the person and experience for which you are grateful.
   c. Describe what emotions you felt during your experience.
   d. Describe what your body felt during that experience.

5. Your facilitator will help you by keeping track of time.

6. When each group is finished, your facilitator may ask volunteers how they feel after the exercise with the entire group. Use one or two words to describe your feelings.

ATTACHMENTS THAT KILL: HOW ADDICTIONS RE-WIRE YOUR BRAIN
BEEPS ATTACHMENT & IDENTITY - MEDICATE TO REGULATE PART 2: HARMFUL DEPENDENCY

TODAY'S LESSON: BEEPS, Attachment and Identity: Medicate to Regulate Part 2: Harmful Dependency

> **Facilitator Note:** Play Session Ten on the Restarting DVD.
> - Ask the class to follow along in their workbooks and take notes as needed.

CLASS NOTES: BEEPS, Attachment & Identity: Medicate to Regulate Part 2: Harmful Dependency

BEEPS
- BEEPS are attachments to Behaviors, Events, Experiences, People or Substances that are used to regulate emotions, increase pleasure or decrease pain.
- Attachments to BEEPS help us medicate – to artificially regulate – positive and negative emotions as well as pain.
- Attachments to BEEPS take the place of secure attachments to God and significant others.

Attachment to beeps is not about an identity rooted in addiction.
- Attachments to BEEPS result when an identity is rooted in pain.
- When there is no way to effectively regulate pain, pleasure or emotions, BEEPS. Attachments hijack the attachment center – and lead to harmful dependency.

Attachment can lead to:
- Healthy interdependence or
- Harmful dependency.

How do attachments to BEEPS develop? How does harmful dependency build?

How do BEEPS attachments develop?
- Now the Lord God had planted a garden in the east, in Eden; ("Eden" means "Pleasure") and there he put the man he had formed. And the Lord God made all kinds of trees grow out of the ground – trees that were pleasing to the eye and good for food.
  Genesis 2: 8-9. NIV, parenthesis added.
- We are created to experience and enjoy pleasure!

Adam and Eve used Eden to cover and hide from pain.
- Then the eyes of both of them were opened, and they realized they were naked; so they sewed fig leaves together and made coverings for themselves. Then the man and his wife heard the sound of the Lord God as He was walking in the garden in the cool of the day and they hid from the Lord God among the trees of the garden.
  Genesis 3: 7-8, NKJV

Adam and Eve used Eden to cover up and hide from:
- God
- Each other
- Painful emotions

They blamed God and each other for their attachment pain (separation from God and each other) and for their ongoing emotional distress.

Broken attachments to God and each other overwhelmed their capacity to handle pain.
- Their level of pain exceeded their level of joy.

ATTACHMENTS THAT KILL: HOW ADDICTIONS RE-WIRE YOUR BRAIN
BEEPS ATTACHMENT & IDENTITY - MEDICATE TO REGULATE PART 2: HARMFUL DEPENDENCY

- They experienced ongoing relational distress and trauma.
- The greater the attachment pain, the less capacity we have for life.

As capacity drops, life becomes more painful.
- I am less able to attach to others in healthy relationships.
- I am stuck in increasing levels of pain.

When I lack joy capacity and get stuck in negative emotions, my attachments with others are a source of ongoing pain.
- Dismissive attachment
- Distracted attachment
- Disorganized attachment

Unresolved attachment pain further diminishes capacity and increases distress:
- Non-secure attachments lead to even greater levels of attachment pain.
- Increasing attachment pain leads to reduced joyful capacity and escalating levels of trauma and chronic distress.
- Rising levels of trauma and chronic distress lead to the development of an identity that is painful.
- My identity is now pain centered.
- I am driven to find relief.

Non-secure attachments and weak identity are the result of:
- Lack of joy capacity.
- Lack of synchronization.
- Getting stuck in pain without the ability to return to joy.
- Level 1 attachment pain.
- An identity that is rooted in pain leads to harmful dependency.

Medicate to regulate

BEEPS
- There are many different types of BEEPS. Examples can include:
- Behaviors: Work
- Events: Thrill Seeking
- Experiences: Sex
- People: Relationships
- Substances: Alcohol

BEEPS hijack the attachment center.
- What we attach to steers us.
- When the emotional control center is hijacked, BEEPS are behind the wheel.
- BEEPS drive us to places of even greater attachment pain.
- BEEPS destroy our lives, homes and relationships.

Attachment strength: the strength of attachments to BEEPS are reflected by:
- Intensity:
  - How strongly the BEEPS changes emotions, pleasure and/or pain.
- Intimacy:
  - How strongly we relate to and rely on BEEPS to medicate emotions, pain and pleasure.
- Exclusivity:
  - The degree to which we focus our time, effort and energy on BEEPS – to the exclusion of other people, things or God.

YOUR NOTES

ATTACHMENTS THAT KILL: HOW ADDICTIONS RE-WIRE YOUR BRAIN
BEEPS ATTACHMENT & IDENTITY - MEDICATE TO REGULATE PART 2: HARMFUL DEPENDENCY

BEEPS attachment strength
The development of an attachment to BEEPS through the stages of intensity, intimacy and exclusivity describes the process by which BEEPS hijack the emotional control center of the brain.
- Intensity:
  - Attachment center and the three non-secure attachment styles
  - Trauma
  - Value systems
  - Control center dysfunction
- Intimacy:
  - Growing BEEPS attachment to regulate emotion, pleasure and pain.
  - Implicit memory (euphoric recall)
  - Acquired value
- Exclusivity:
  - Alterations in dopamine receptors
  - Craving
  - Resistant to other attachments and stimuli
  - Structural changes in the control center
- Harmful dependency:
  - Tolerance and withdrawal
  - Relationship destruction
  - Specific BEEPS disease process
  - Increasing breakdown of the control center
  - Illness, high risk behaviors
  - Death

Intensity and trauma
- The neurological and behavioral pathways for addictive behaviors are forged during infancy and childhood through repeated exposure to relational trauma. Once the individual discovers that substance use and related behaviors can expedite and mimic the chemical process that leads to immediate relief from psychic pain, the process shifts to a set of maladaptive addictive behaviors.... Addictive behaviors share the same pathways in the brain with trauma-based behaviors. Dr. Joel Porter, 2002.
- This same relationship between trauma and addictive behaviors is further illustrated in Dr. Allan Schore's work "Affect Dysregulation and Disorders of the Self."

Intensity, trauma and monkeys:
- After socialization, dominant (untraumatized) monkeys had 20% more volume ratio for D2 dopamine receptors.
- D2 did not predict social order, but predicted cocaine usage.
- Subordinate monkeys self-administered cocaine at higher rates than dominant.
- Subordinate monkeys were more sensitive to the reinforcing effects of cocaine than dominant.
- Dominant monkeys were initially protected from the reinforcing effects of cocaine, but over time, they lost the increased volume of dopamine receptors.

Intimacy, acquired value and memory:
- "Associated memories are laid down that change the emotional value of drugs that created deeply ingrained behavioral responses to those cues."
  - Laura Helmuth, Science, Nov. 2, 2001, quoting Steve Hyman, Director of the National Institute of Mental Health.
- "Non-conscious memories are more likely to underlie the compulsive aspect of addiction and the cravings that lead to relapse. For instance, the paraphernalia of drug

ATTACHMENTS THAT KILL: HOW ADDICTIONS RE-WIRE YOUR BRAIN
BEEPS ATTACHMENT & IDENTITY - MEDICATE TO REGULATE PART 2: HARMFUL DEPENDENCY

use – crack pipes, syringes, the sound of ice tinkling in a glass full of scotch – can act as cues that induce craving much like the sound of a bell caused Pavlov's dogs to salivate."

> Laura Helmuth, Science, Nov. 2, 2001, quoting Terry Robinson, University of Michigan.

Exclusivity, D2 receptors and monkeys:
- Cocaine use alters D2 receptor functioning.
  - In humans, even after 4 months abstinence. (The study stopped at 4 months, because everyone relapsed!)
  - In monkeys, even after 7 months.
  - Chronic exposure resulted in persistent reductions in D2 receptor densities.
  - In cocaine using monkeys, receptor binding 20% lower. Controls had excellent uptake in basal ganglia.
  > Nader and Czoty, "PET Imaging of Dopamine D2 Receptors in Monkey Models of Cocaine Abuse: Genetic Predisposition Versus Environmental Modulation." American Journal of Psychiatry, 162:8, August. 2005.
- Alcoholics have the same issue in the reward pathway.
  > Heinz, et al., "Correlation Between Dopamine D2 Receptors in the Ventral Striatum and Central Process of Alcohol Cues and Craving." American Journal of Psychiatry 2004; 161:1783-1789.

Why is D2 reduction important?
- Impairment in dopamine sensitivity means:
  - The person recovering from BEEPS experiences less pleasure in normal life.
  - Other stimuli – even healthy ones – are not as attractive as the BEEPS.
  - Dopamine processing has been altered to respond primarily to BEEPS.
  > Franken, I. H. Drug Craving and Addiction: Integrating Psychological and Neuropsychopharmacological Approaches. Prog. Neuropsychopharmocological Biologic Psychiatry. 2003 June; 27(4):563-79.
- This makes the BEEPS relationship even more exclusive.
- **BEEPS is a jealous lover!**

Disruption of the control center
The following studies are not discussed on the video, but are included here for your review.
- Numerous studies suggest alterations in the functions of the basal ganglia and thalamus, amygdala, cingulate cortex, and the orbitoprefrontal cortex:
  - "These alterations suggest that during craving, activity in reward pathways increases, while cognitive control decreases."
  - "These may be a consequence of a pre-existent vulnerability to addictive behavior."
  > "Substance Use Disorders and the Orbitofrontal Cortex." British Journal of Psychiatry, 2005. 187, 209-220.
- Other studies suggest:
  - Executive dysfunction in the right prefrontal cortex and cingulate and over-reliance on the left hemisphere of the brain to complete tasks.
  - This makes it hard to inhibit behavior.
  - Addiction deregulates executive functioning.
  - Personality changes.
  > Hester & Garavan. "Executive Dysfunction in Cocaine Addiction: Evidence for Discordant Frontal, Cingulate and Cerebellar Activity." The Journal of Neuroscience, December 8, 2004. 24(49); 11017-11022.

ATTACHMENTS THAT KILL: HOW ADDICTIONS RE-WIRE YOUR BRAIN
BEEPS ATTACHMENT & IDENTITY - MEDICATE TO REGULATE PART 2: HARMFUL DEPENDENCY

Heinz, et al. "Correlation Between Dopamine D2 Receptors in the Ventral Striatum and Central Processing of Alcohol Cues and Craving." American Journal of Psychiatry 2004; 161:1783-1789.

Since BEEPS are about a painful identity, effective recovery must:
- Be relational.
- Recognize and identify both beeps and pain.
- Address both beeps and the painful identity.
- Develop secure relationships with others that are empowered by joy.
- Change my identity!

Sobriety is the primary focus of self-help and Twelve Step recovery groups.
- Helping participants remain abstinent from life-controlling and destructive addictions is the primary goal of most Twelve Step and self-help groups.
- Since addictions destroy lives, family and relationships, sobriety is essential.
- The Twelve Steps can help provide an important blueprint for sobriety.

The goals of thriving are deeper:
- Thriving is a relational program that is based on cutting-edge research from "The Decade of the Brain."
- Thriving teaches participants the joy and relationship-building skills they need to help the brain heal from the devastating effects of unhealthy attachments and traumas.
- Thriving promotes sobriety – but much, much more.

Thriving leads to identity change and the growth of healing community.
- As the brain becomes empowered by joy, Thriving participants are able to connect to others in ways that are mutually life giving.
- A new joyful identity develops that leads to mutually satisfying relationships – and the growth of ongoing maturity.
- Life-giving and joyful community allows all members to grow together.

Thriving and Steps 8 & 9
- Step 8: Made a list of all persons we had harmed, and became willing to make amends to them all.
- Step 9: Made direct amends to such people wherever possible, except when to do so would injure them or others.

BEEPS recovery is about relationship.
- When we are attached to BEEPS, we use people, places and things to regulate pain.
- An essential task for recovery is making amends to others that we have harmed through BEEPS.
- This can help us restore relationships and build healthy attachments with others.

Steps 8 and 9 and identity:
- Accepting responsibility for the harm my BEEPS attachments have caused is only the beginning.
- To change my identity, I must develop and maintain secure and joyful attachments with others.
- Steps 8 & 9 help me develop these new and life-giving relationships.

ATTACHMENTS THAT KILL: HOW ADDICTIONS RE-WIRE YOUR BRAIN
BEEPS ATTACHMENT & IDENTITY - MEDICATE TO REGULATE PART 2: HARMFUL DEPENDENCY

EXERCISE: TELLING A LEVEL 4 ATTACHMENT TO BEEPS STORY
15 Minutes

Facilitator Note: This exercise is designed to help participants apply and review the concepts they have just learned about attachments to BEEPS by telling Level 4 stories. In previous lessons, we learned that Level 4 stories are non-verbal exercises that allow the right hemisphere of the brain to express itself without having to use words. Participants tell Level 4 stories by using facial expressions, body language and movement.

Level 4 stories can be a lot of fun for groups. It may help to describe Level 4 stories as an opportunity to "Go to Hollywood," because it gives everyone a chance to try out their acting skills. You will need to review the characteristics of a Level 4 story with your group. In this exercise, participants will use their non-verbal communication skills to answer the question, "What do attachments to BEEPS look like?"

Please keep two things in mind as you facilitate this exercise. First, be aware that attachments to BEEPS can be a very painful topic of discussion. Telling Level 4 stories – instead of Level 4+ stories – can help reduce the distress and anxiety that participants may experience with this topic. Telling a Level 4 story can help participants better understand what attachments to BEEPS look like, without unnecessarily raising their level of pain.

Second, be aware that this week's lesson discusses the subject of euphoric recall and BEEPS in detail. It is possible that this discussion will trigger feelings and memories of euphoric recall in participants who have had intense and intimate relationships with BEEPS. Some participants may also feel a great deal of shame or disgust when they discuss euphoric recall.

Two aspects of this exercise can help participants deal with euphoric recall. First, this exercise emphasizes the terribly destructive emotional pain caused by attachments to BEEPS. This reminds participants that even though early use of BEEPS may have been intensely pleasurable, attachments to BEEPS later resulted in tremendous pain. Second, you can synchronize with participants who are feeling ashamed of their euphoric recall by sharing a Level 4+ story about a time when you experienced euphoric recall – and how you overcame it. Prepare your 4+ story in advance, and make sure that the story is not too intense! You will have 3 minutes to tell your story. It is not necessary for the group to give you feedback about your story.

It is helpful to prepare your group to tell their Level 4 stories by first asking them to describe what the pain of attachments to BEEPS feels like. Volunteers may answer by using one or two words to describe BEEPS attachments. You can also prepare participants by telling your own Level 4 story in which you describe what BEEPS attachments look like. When you have finished, volunteers will be ready to begin telling their Level 4 stories.

YOUR NOTES

1. It is not necessary to break into small groups for this exercise.

2. Your facilitator will review the characteristics of a Level 4 story with you.
    a. Level 4 stories are non-verbal stories.
    b. Level 4 stories express the experiences, feelings, and sensations of the right hemisphere, without using words from the left hemisphere of the brain to describe them.
    c. In Level 4 stories, participants act out the story and emotions they are describing using only facial expression, body language, movement or non-verbal interactions with others.

ATTACHMENTS THAT KILL: HOW ADDICTIONS RE-WIRE YOUR BRAIN
BEEPS ATTACHMENT & IDENTITY - MEDICATE TO REGULATE PART 2: HARMFUL DEPENDENCY

YOUR NOTES

3. Your facilitator will take a few minutes to talk with you about euphoric recall.
   a. Since this lesson discussed attachments to BEEPS and euphoric recall in detail, it is very normal that some of you may be experiencing euphoric recall about past use of BEEPS.
   b. Euphoric recall is a neurochemical process triggered by conscious or sub-concious memories of the pleasure we felt when we used BEEPS.
   c. Experiencing euphoric recall is not shameful. Learning to overcome an experience of euphoric recall is a normal part of recovery.
   d. Your facilitator will share a Level 4+ story with you about a time in which he/she experienced – and overcame – euphoric recall.

4. When your facilitator's Level 4+ story about euphoric recall is complete, your facilitator will ask volunteers to share one-word descriptions of what attachments to BEEPS feel like.

5. Your facilitator will tell a Level 4 BEEPS Attachment Story for the entire group that describes what BEEPS attachments look like.

6. Volunteers have the opportunity to tell a Level 4 story about what attachments to BEEPS look like.
   a. Remember to tell these stories using only facial expression, body language, or movement.
   b. Have fun with this! You are, "Going to Hollywood."

7. Your facilitator will help you by keeping track of time.

EXERCISE: RELAXING WITH JESUS - THE IMMANUEL PROCESS
25 Minutes

Facilitator Note: This exercise combines a portion of the breathing and relaxation exercises we learned in week 2 with the Immanuel Process. This exercise helps participants relax, experience the presence of Jesus and build joy and bonds as volunteers share their experience with their small group. It will be helpful for you to prepare for this exercise by reviewing the instructions for the Immanuel Process from Week 7.

In Week 2 of Restarting, we learned that when we are distressed, we tend to take rapid, shallow breaths. By paying attention to our breathing – and learning to breathe deeply, we are making sure that our brain is receiving enough oxygen. We are also activating the right orbital prefrontal cortex of our brain. Practicing deep breathing exercises can also help us think through our options when we are distressed, and avoid making poor decisions made in hasty reactions to stress. They can also help us to relax and improve our ability to perceive the presence of Jesus with us.

In Week 7, we learned and experienced a simple Immanuel Process exercise. We learned that the name "Immanuel" means "God with us," and is one of the names that is used to describe Jesus in the Old and New Testaments. The Immanuel Process is an exercise that is designed to help participants recognize the presence of Jesus in their lives.

Though Jesus has promised to be with us always, (Matt 28:20), we are not always aware that He is present with us. Like the disciples on the Emmaus Road, (Luke 24:13-32) it is

ATTACHMENTS THAT KILL: HOW ADDICTIONS RE-WIRE YOUR BRAIN
BEEPS ATTACHMENT & IDENTITY - MEDICATE TO REGULATE PART 2: HARMFUL DEPENDENCY

possible for Jesus to be with us – but for us to not perceive His presence. The Immanuel Process is based upon the scriptural truth that Jesus is always with us – and that He can open the eyes of our heart so that we can perceive His presence with us. Our life will forever change as we learn to trust and rely on the comforting presence, joy and ever-present love of the One who is with us.

The Immanuel Process can be an important part of recovery from attachments to BEEPS and the trauma of euphoric recall. Just as memories of euphoric recall or attachments to BEEPS can affect our lives in the present, memories of joy with Jesus can also powerfully affect our lives today. As we become intentional about recalling our experiences with Jesus, our memories of those moments can lay a new foundation for relational recovery from trauma. These joyful encounters with Jesus can help us build new joyful capacity.

Remembering and meditating on joyful moments with Jesus helps build enough capacity so that He is able to lead us through areas of life that do not feel peaceful. These non-peaceful moments can include craving, euphoric recall and shame about our attachments to BEEPS. He literally builds enough capacity in us so that we are able to heal – and overcome attachments to BEEPS – by perceiving His presence in difficult areas of life.

One of the most devastating aspects of attachments to BEEPS is that we feel alone, isolated and cut off from others in our pain. Our feelings of anger, shame, disgust, fear, sadness and hopeless despair about our attachments to BEEPS can be overwhelming. When we are able to perceive that Jesus loves us and is glad to be with us – even when we feel these negative emotions – we receive comfort, healing and a sense of being deeply connected with Jesus. We learn that we are never alone.

In this week's Immanuel Process exercise, participants will be asked to remember a time or experience in which they felt that Jesus was very near to them. This can be described as a "peak experience" with Jesus, in which they were unusually aware of His presence. They will be asked to remember the details of the experience, and what their emotions and body felt like when they were with him. Participants are encouraged to reflect on this experience and to enjoy the presence of Jesus.

After participants have had time to reflect and enjoy the presence of Jesus, participants will be invited to ask Jesus a few simple questions such as: "Jesus, do you love me? Are you glad to be with me? Is there anything you would like to say to me now? Is there anything you want me to do now?" In this portion of the exercise, the facilitator may quietly remind participants of these questions. Participants may ask these questions silently, and listen quietly for the answers.

After participants have had time to reflect on their experience with Jesus, they will have opportunity to share about their experience in a small group. Sharing about experiences with Jesus builds individual and group capacity.

As mentioned in previous weeks, please keep in mind that some participants may not be able to describe a "peak experience" or time in which they felt particularly close with Jesus. This may be due to a variety of factors. Some may have never asked Jesus to be part of their life, and as a result, have had no real awareness of His presence. Others may have experienced severe wounding or trauma, which has made it difficult for them to remember a time in which they felt very close to Jesus. In some cases, participants may have too much fear to engage in this process – or have just never learned to recognize the presence of Jesus. Some will have attachment problems.

YOUR NOTES

ATTACHMENTS THAT KILL: HOW ADDICTIONS RE-WIRE YOUR BRAIN
BEEPS ATTACHMENT & IDENTITY - MEDICATE TO REGULATE PART 2: HARMFUL DEPENDENCY

> It is important that you explain these possible obstacles before the exercise begins. It is also important that everyone, regardless of personal experience, can participate as active listeners in the small group process that is part of this exercise. Sometimes, listening as another person describes a joyful and meaningful encounter with Jesus can help create a desire for a relationship with Jesus in someone who does not yet know Him. Descriptions of joyful and life giving encounters with Jesus can help reduce fear in those who are fearful, and can also provide useful examples of what the presence of Jesus feels like for those who have never learned to recognize Him. Finally, Jesus knows that someone may be in too much pain from trauma - or experiencing the blockages caused by trauma – to easily perceive His presence. It is important to reassure these participants that Jesus will provide other people to help provide what they need to break through these barriers. Everyone, regardless of their ability to perceive the presence of Jesus can benefit from the small group sharing that is part of this exercise. Joy bonds will build as joyful stories about Jesus are shared.
>
> Finally, please keep in mind that a genuine experience or encounter with Jesus will always be consistent with the character and nature of Jesus as revealed in the Scripture.

1. Break into small groups of 3-5 people.

2. For the first part of this exercise, you are welcome to find a comfortable position in which you can rest and relax. You may remain in your chair, sit or lie down on the floor, stand – or whatever feels most comfortable to you. (5-7 Minutes)

3. Place your hand over your stomach. Take such a deep breath that you feel your stomach expand as you breathe. Follow your facilitator's instructions as you breathe deeply for a few moments.
   a. When we are stressed, we tend to take rapid shallow breaths. By learning deep breathing exercises and paying attention to what our bodies are doing, we are making sure that our brain is receiving enough oxygen, and we are activating the right orbital prefrontal cortex of our brain.
   b. Practicing deep breathing exercises can also help us think through our options when we are distressed, and avoid making poor decisions made in hasty reactions to stress.
   c. Both of these are helpful in overcoming cravings and BEEPS attachments. They can also help us to relax and improve our ability to perceive the presence of Jesus with us.

4. As you continue to breathe deeply and relax, your facilitator will share with you a time when he/she experienced the presence of God in a way that was meaningful and memorable. He/she will describe:
   a. What happened in the experience he/she is describing.
   b. The emotions he/she felt when he/she was with Jesus.
   c. What his/her body felt like when he/she was with Jesus.
   d. What he/she did when he/se experienced His presence.

5. When the story is complete, your facilitator will remind you to continue to breathe deeply.

6. Your facilitator will also explain the reasons that some people may have difficulty experiencing or perceiving the presence of Jesus. (2 Minutes)
   a. Some participants may not be able to describe a "peak experience" or time in which they felt particularly close with Jesus. This may be due to a variety of

ATTACHMENTS THAT KILL: HOW ADDICTIONS RE-WIRE YOUR BRAIN
BEEPS ATTACHMENT & IDENTITY - MEDICATE TO REGULATE PART 2: HARMFUL DEPENDENCY

YOUR NOTES

factors, including the presence of exceptionally severe trauma that has formed blockages that keep them from perceiving His presence. These participants can be encouraged that Jesus often wants to help them by bringing other people into their life that can help them resolve these blockages.

b. Some may have never asked Jesus to be part of their life, and as a result, have had no real awareness of His presence. It may be appropriate to ask these participants if they would like to invite Jesus to help them perceive His presence.

c. Some participants may experience strong fear that keeps them from perceiving Jesus' presence – or may never have learned to recognize the presence of Jesus.

d. All participants – regardless of their ability to perceive the presence of Jesus – are encouraged to continue with their deep breathing and relaxation exercises throughout the entire exercise. They are also invited to participate in the entire Immanuel Process exercise to whatever extent they feel comfortable.

7. Your facilitator will again remind you to continue to breathe deeply.

8. Your facilitator will invite you to close your eyes, and ask Jesus to help you remember a time when you felt very close to Him. As your eyes are closed, your facilitator may help you by quietly asking the questions listed below. You do not need to answer these questions aloud; the questions are only to help you focus on the memory of your experience with Jesus. Your facilitator will help you by keeping track of time during this portion of the exercise and let you know when it is time to open your eyes. (3 Minutes)
   a. What is happening in the experience you are remembering?
   b. What emotions are you feeling?
   c. What does your body feel like when you are with Jesus?
   d. What are you doing in that memory?
   e. How does it feel to be with Jesus?

9. After you have had the time to reflect on this experience with Jesus, you may ask Jesus a series of questions. As before, your facilitator may help you by quietly reminding you of these questions. You do not need to answer these questions aloud. You may ask these questions silently, and wait to perceive a response. These can include questions like: (3 Minutes)
   a. Jesus, do you love me?
   b. Are you glad to be with me?
   c. Is there anything you would like to say to me now?
   d. Is there anything you want me to do now?

10. Your facilitator will help you by keeping track of time during this portion of the exercise, and let you know when it is time to open your eyes.

11. After you open your eyes, please gather in your small groups, and volunteers can begin to take turns sharing about their experience for 2 minutes. Your facilitator will help you keep track of time as you share. Remember to stay relational by making eye contact as you describe:
    a. The experience with Jesus you just remembered.
    b. The emotions you felt in the memory.
    c. What your body felt like.
    d. What you did when you felt the presence of Jesus.
    e. How it feels to remember this experience with Jesus.

ATTACHMENTS THAT KILL: HOW ADDICTIONS RE-WIRE YOUR BRAIN
BEEPS ATTACHMENT & IDENTITY - MEDICATE TO REGULATE PART 2: HARMFUL DEPENDENCY

YOUR NOTES

12. When each participant has had the opportunity to share their experience with their small group, your facilitator may ask volunteers to describe what it feels like to experience the presence of Jesus with the entire group. Use one or two words to describe your feelings. (1-2 Minutes)

CLOSE THE GROUP WITH PRAYER

ATTACHMENTS THAT KILL: HOW ADDICTIONS RE-WIRE YOUR BRAIN
BEEPS ATTACHMENT & IDENTITY - MEDICATE TO REGULATE PART 2: HARMFUL DEPENDENCY

QUESTIONS FOR FURTHER DISCUSSION OR FOLLOW-UP

1. How can covering up, hiding or denial of our problems lead to attachment pain? How has your own covering, hiding and denial increased your level of attachment pain?

2. Have you ever blamed other people, places or things for problems and pain that are your own responsibility? Have you ever blamed these people, places or things for your own attachments to BEEPS? Explain.

3. Do you believe that a significant portion of your identity has been pain-centered? Explain. How has this affected your life?

4. Have attachments to BEEPS taken your life to places of even greater pain? What happened? List at least 3 of these painful places.

5. What is the intensity stage of attachments to BEEPS? Why is intensity so important in the development of attachments to BEEPS?

6. Why is it so easy for BEEPS to feel so intensely pleasurable when our control center is not functioning effectively?

7. How do you define the intimacy stage of attachment to BEEPS? How does this lead to stronger attachments to BEEPS?

8. What is euphoric recall? Why is it such an important part of the development of attachment to BEEPS? Why is it so important in relapse? Has it ever been a part of your own BEEPS relapse?

9. What is acquired value? Why do things associated with our use of BEEPS become important relapse triggers?

10. How do you define the exclusivity stage of attachments to BEEPS?

11. What is craving? Why are BEEPS such a jealous lover?

12. What are the characteristics of the harmful dependency stage of attachments to BEEPS?

13. Why is it essential for you to have a change of identity in recovery?

14. List 5 essential characteristics of an effective trauma and BEEPS recovery program.

15. Why do you need a joyful recovery community? Where is your own joyful recovery community?

16. Why are Steps 8 and 9 important for relational recovery?

17. Describe your experience with the Immanuel Process exercise this week.

ATTACHMENTS THAT KILL: HOW ADDICTIONS RE-WIRE YOUR BRAIN
BEEPS ATTACHMENT & IDENTITY - MEDICATE TO REGULATE PART 2: HARMFUL DEPENDENCY

OPTIONAL 12-STEP QUESTIONS

1. What do Steps 8 and 9, and the word "amends" mean to you? Why are these important for your recovery?

2. Has your identity become largely rooted in pain? List 3 characteristics of your painful identity that you would like to change in recovery.

3. Denying, covering up or hiding our problems and attachments to BEEPS – and blaming them on other people, places and things – are characteristics of an identity that is rooted in pain.
   a. Make a list of as many problems and attachments to BEEPS that you tried to cover up, hide or deny as you can recall. How did you try to hide, cover up or deny these issues? Be as specific as you can.
   b. Make a list of as many people, places and things you blamed for your problems and attachments to BEEPS as you can recall. What problems did you blame on each of these? Be as specific as you can.

4. Did covering up, hiding, denial and blaming increase your own level of attachment pain? How did you handle this increased pain?

5. Who were the people that were affected by the hiding, covering up, denial and blaming that you listed in question 3? How did your actions affect each of them? Be specific.

6. As our attachments with BEEPS became more intimate and exclusive, we had less time, attention, effort and resources for relationships with those who cared about us the most. Make a list of the people who were most affected as our time, attention, effort and resources became increasingly devoted to BEEPS. Describe how your attachments to BEEPS affected each one. Be specific.

7. Are there other people that your attachments to BEEPS harmed that you have not listed yet? Who are these people, and how did your BEEPS attachments hurt them?

8. Why is it so important to make amends to those we have harmed?

9. Are you willing to make amends to the people you've harmed?
   a. Make a list of the people you've harmed and to whom you are willing to make amends. List the specific amends you would like to make.
   b. Make a list of the people you've harmed – but to whom you don't want to make amends. What do you need to become willing?

10. Step 9 says that whenever possible, we should make direct amends to all those we've harmed – except when to do so would injure them or others. Are there people on your list that would be harmed if you tried to make amends?

11. How can a joyful community help you develop a new identity – and build the capacity to make amends to others?

12. What are the 5 characteristics of an effective recovery program?

13. Why do you need a joyful community to recover from trauma and attachments to BEEPS?

14. What resources do you need to help you work on Steps 8 and 9? What are they, and where can you find them?

11 RECOVERING OUR LOST IDENTITY
MATURITY AND CAPACITY PART 1: WHAT IS MATURITY?

OPEN THE GROUP

YOUR NOTES

- Ask for a volunteer to open the group in prayer.

EXERCISE: A NEW BEGINNING *10 Minutes*

Facilitator Note: The purpose of this exercise is to help participants begin to think about the kind of future they would like in recovery from trauma and attachments to BEEPS.

Last week's material focused on helping participants recognize the overwhelming devastation that a painful identity, BEEPS attachments and harmful dependency can bring to life. This recognition, though painful, is an important part of the recovery process. Just as important, however, is the need to begin to think about what a new life in recovery might be like. Recovery is the journey in which we are empowered to discover a new life and recover our true identity. It is a completely new beginning. Helping participants develop vision and hope for their new future is an essential task for recovery.

This exercise invites participants to start asking the question, "What do I want my new life in recovery to look like?" Participants will list three things that they hope will characterize their new life, and have the opportunity to share these in a small group. You can help participants begin to answer this question by sharing three characteristics that describe your life in recovery.

1. Break into small groups of 3-5 people.

2. Your facilitator will share with you that:
   a. Recovery is a journey in which we are empowered to discover a new life – and recover our true identity.
   b. It is a journey of hope, and a new beginning.
   c. It is important to begin to think about what our new life in recovery can be like.

3. Your facilitator will share with you either:
   a. Three characteristics that describe what their life is like now that they are in recovery.
   b. Three characteristics that describe what they hope their life will be like in recovery.

4. Your facilitator will ask you the question, "What do you want your life in recovery to look like?" Take a few minutes to ask yourself this question, and then write down three things that you hope will characterize your new life in recovery.

   Characteristic 1:_____

   Characteristic 2:_____

   Characteristic 3:_____

RECOVERING OUR LOST IDENTITY
MATURITY AND CAPACITY PART 1: WHAT IS MATURITY?

YOUR NOTES

5. Your facilitator will let you know when volunteers can begin sharing their answers with their small group. You will each have 2 minutes to share.
    a. Remember to make eye contact as you share your answers.
    b. Remember to listen as each person shares, and do not offer feedback or advice.

6. Your facilitator will help you by keeping track of time for you.

TODAY'S LESSON: Maturity and Capacity Part 1: What is Maturity?

Facilitator Note: Play Session Eleven on the Restarting DVD.
• Ask the class to follow along in their workbooks, and take notes as needed.

CLASS NOTES: Maturity and Capacity Part 1: What is Maturity?

So what is maturity?
- What does it look like?
- How do you know it when you see it?

Growth and maturity are God's ideas!
- Then God blessed them, and God said to them, "Be fruitful and multiply; fill the earth and subdue it…" Genesis 1: 28, NKJV

He created us to need others to grow into full maturity.
- Without others, it is impossible for us to mature.

We are not born fully mature, physically or spiritually

Maturity is a lifetime journey:
- Until we're all moving rhythmically and easily with each other, efficient and graceful in response to God's Son, fully mature adults, fully developed without and within, fully alive like Christ. Ephesians 4:11-13 The Message.

Maturity is not based on physical age.

Physical age is relevant
- But not the only determining factor for defining maturity.

A five year old cannot be an elder
- Although a fifty year old can be stuck at an infant level of maturity.

Maturing means reaching our God given potential.

We mature when we maximize our identity.

We use our skills and talents effectively.

Maturity is growing to the full capacity of our individual designs.

Maturity is not a spiritual gift nor is it a by-product of salvation.

Maturity does not fall from heaven.
- Maturity is a gift we give each other.

RECOVERING OUR LOST IDENTITY
MATURITY AND CAPACITY PART 1: WHAT IS MATURITY?

YOUR NOTES

Maturity does not grow on trees.
- We grow maturity ourselves through hard work.

Maturity is the human task:
- Redemption is God's task:
  - Healing
  - Deliverance
  - Salvation
  - Sanctification

Maturing means we receive before we give.

Maturity is something we work on our entire lives.
- Some are just a little further along than others!

Maturing never ends or finishes.
- We never stop needing other people.

Family and community help us mature.

Life in community is best when people have life-giving relationships with those in all the other stages of life.

Maturing doesn't give us more value.
- As for the man who is weak in faith, welcome him, but not for disputes over opinions. One believes he may eat anything, while the weak man eats only vegetables. Let not him who eats despise him who abstains, and let not him who abstains pass judgment on him who eats; for God has welcomed him. Romans 14: 1-3, RSV

Maturing is valuable
- And his gifts were that some should be apostles, some prophets, some evangelists, some pastors and teachers, to equip the saints for the work of ministry, for building up the body of Christ, until we all attain to the unity of the faith and of the knowledge of the Son of God, to mature manhood, to the measure of the stature of the fullness of Christ; so that we may no longer be children, tossed to and fro and carried about with every wind of doctrine, by the cunning of men, by their craftiness in deceitful wiles. Rather, speaking the truth in love, we are to grow up in every way into him who is the head, into Christ. Ephesians 4:11-15, RSV.

How do we build capacity and maturity?

Attachments are the building blocks for mature and healthy brains.
- Healthy attachments to others who are empowered by joy create healthy brains that can regulate emotions, pleasure and pain.
- Unhealthy attachments to others who are not empowered by joy create unhealthy brains that do not effectively regulate emotions, pleasure and pain.

Secure attachment results from high joy capacity and synchronized bonds.
- My identity is joyful, strong and secure.
- This allows me to form secure bonds with others.

The brain has two hemispheres that are different:
- Left hemisphere: naming and explaining
- Right hemisphere: knowing and experience

RECOVERING OUR LOST IDENTITY
MATURITY AND CAPACITY PART 1: WHAT IS MATURITY?

Building joy and joy capacity help build maturity.
- Increasing capacity helps develop identity that is strong – even when facing Increasing distress.
- Maturity grows.

I mature in rhythms of joy and quiet together that create secure attachments and an identity that is joyful, secure and strong.

When others are glad to be with us when we are distressed:
- I can learn to return to joy from negative emotions.
- My attachments and bonds remain secure.
- I can act like myself, even when I'm upset.
- I learn this skill in the second year of life.
- These allow secure attachments to grow, even when I'm distressed or upset.
- My individual and group identity is strengthened, and this helps me grow in maturity through pain!

Secure attachments with a strong, joyful individual and group identity build healthy interdependence and ongoing maturity.

BEEPS
- Pseudo joy can produce the appearance of capacity and maturity.
- But will fail under stress.

BEEPS and pseudo joy will always result in ongoing and chronic immaturity.

Immaturity is a level 4 problem in the emotional control center.
- BEEPS are the result of a catastrophic failure to reach adult maturity – and keep us stuck in immaturity!

The Twelve Steps can help us address the pain and trauma of the BEEPS cycle:
- Relationship with God
  - Steps 1, 2, 3 and 11.
- Relationship with Self
  - Steps 4, 5, 6, 7 and 10.
- Relationship with Others
  - Steps 8, 9, and 12.
- When these relationships grow in balance, our recovery will also remain balanced.
- Without growth in all 3 of these relationships, recovery will be out of balance, and will not stand.
- Steps 10, 11 & 12 are called "maintenance steps" and can help produce ongoing sobriety & maturity.

Steps 10 – 12: maintaining and maturing
- Step 10: self
  - Continued to take personal inventory and when we were wrong, promptly admitted it.
- Step 11: God
  - Sought through prayer and meditation to improve our conscious contact with God as we understood Him, praying only for the knowledge of His will for us and the power to carry that out.
- Step 12: others
  - Having had a spiritual awakening as a result of these steps, we tried to carry this message to alcoholics, and to practice these principles in all our affairs.

RECOVERING OUR LOST IDENTITY
MATURITY AND CAPACITY PART 1: WHAT IS MATURITY?

YOUR NOTES

EXERCISE: A SCRIPTURE MEDITATION - TALKING TO JESUS *40 Minutes*

Facilitator Note: For the past several weeks, participants have been learning to perceive the presence of Jesus through the Immanuel Process. Through a series of progressive weekly exercises, participants have learned to experience and recognize the presence of Jesus in peaceful and non-peaceful areas of life, and to listen as Jesus has answered simple questions. Today's exercise builds upon these previous experiences to help participants encounter, perceive and listen to Jesus through a simple Scripture meditation exercise.

In this exercise, participants will learn to reflect on a passage of scripture, and actively dialogue with Jesus about it. They will also learn to journal as they record the impressions they have from their conversation with Jesus. This empowering and interactive scripture meditation builds capacity, and helps participants practice their skills at perceiving the presence of Jesus. Scriptures become alive and meaningful as participants discover that Jesus is with them to help them understand and apply what they are reading.

Scripture meditation, without the presence of Jesus, rapidly becomes a source of frustration and futility. Without His help in understanding and applying the contents and principles of scripture to daily life, Bible reading can become a dry, left-brained, intellectual process. Information gathering – not Life Formation – tends to be the result of this kind of approach. To those in recovery from trauma and BEEPS, this type of information gathering approach to scripture fails utterly, and becomes counter-productive.

Life-formation is possible when we have an experienced-based encounter with Jesus as we read the scriptures. Experiencing His presence as He helps us understand His words transforms scripture study into a process that affects both the left and right hemispheres of the brain. Life-formation, joy-bonds and healing are the result. This is the type of encounter with Jesus that today's exercise is designed to facilitate.

As you facilitate this exercise, please keep in mind that participants will have a diversity of understanding and familiarity with the scriptures. It is not likely that many will have ever experienced an exercise like this before. Some may have never even tried to study the scriptures; others may have devoted considerable attention to them.

To facilitate this exercise, choose one of the scriptures listed on the Scripture Meditation Worksheet in your workbook. You will also need a pen or pencil to record your impressions as you dialogue with Jesus about the scripture you choose. It is not necessary for you to prepare a detailed Bible study of this passage. In fact, it is better that you do not study this passage ahead of time. The focus of this exercise is interacting with Jesus about what He would like you to learn from the passage – not about what you already know about the passage.

To begin this exercise, ask participants to locate the Scripture Meditation Worksheet in their workbook. It is important that you emphasize that this exercise is an extension of the Immanuel Process that they have been learning for several weeks. Talking with God about scripture is a dynamic, two-way process that helps us experience the pres-ence of Jesus in a way that is life giving. The focus of this exercise is on experiencing the presence of Jesus in a conversation with Him about scripture. The purpose of the exercise is life formation – not an information or data gathering process.

On the worksheet, you will notice that there is a scripture that reads, "And unto Enoch was born Irad: and Irad begat Mehujael: and Mehujael begat Methusael: and Methusael begat Lamech." Genesis 4:18, KJV. Although it is scripture, participants who have

RECOVERING OUR LOST IDENTITY
MATURITY AND CAPACITY PART 1: WHAT IS MATURITY?

never read or studied the Bible will probably have a great deal of trouble working up any kind of enthusiasm for a study of this passage. This is not a good place to start, and it is helpful to point this out to participants.

Next, point out to participants the other passages of scripture on the worksheet. You will need to choose one of these passages of scripture to demonstrate this exercise for participants. Find a comfortable place to sit as you lead this exercise. To demonstrate the exercise:
- Read the passage of scripture aloud.
- If any particular part of that passage catches your attention, stop and ask Jesus aloud what He would like you to know or understand about it.
- If nothing in the passage catches your attention, wait until you finish reading it and then ask Jesus aloud what He would like you to know or understand about it
- Stop, listen and pay attention for any impression or thought that may come to mind. Repeat these out loud to the entire group.
- Record your impressions on the worksheet
- Continue to dialogue with Jesus about the passage, or your impressions. Repeat your questions and impressions aloud as you continue to record them on your worksheet.
- When you have finished your conversation, thank Jesus, or tell Him about an aspect of your time with Him that you particularly appreciated.

Please notice that while doing this exercise, you need to pay attention to the thoughts or impressions that may come to mind as you interact with Jesus. Many of us experience His presence in different ways. Sometimes, we become aware of new thoughts as we dialogue with Him. Sometimes, we discover that we have a new picture in our minds that is based on the scripture, or on our interactions with Him. Sometimes, we simply sense, feel and know Jesus' presence with us. For that reason, it is more useful to describe the word "impressions" to describe our dialogue with Jesus. It is not necessary to use terminology like, "Thus saith the Lord," "God says" to describe our impressions.

After you have modeled this exercise for participants, it is their turn to try the exercise. Ask participants to break down into small groups of 3-5 people. When they are in small groups, you may encourage them to find a position that will be comfortable to them for the next few minutes. They may remain in their seats, sit on the floor, stand or lie down – whatever is comfortable for them. When they are settled, ask participants to choose one of the passages of scripture listed on the worksheet. They will have 10 minutes to silently dialogue with Jesus about the passage of scripture and record their impressions on their worksheet.

When participants have finished recording their dialogue with Jesus, volunteers will have the opportunity to share their impressions and experience in small group. Each person will have 2 minutes to share. At the conclusion of the exercise, volunteers may describe their experience in one or two words with the entire group.

1. It is not necessary to break into small groups for the first part of this exercise.

2. Locate the Scripture Meditation Worksheet in your workbook. Listen as your facilitator explains the purpose of this exercise.
   a. This exercise is similar to the Immanuel Process that we have already learned.
   b. The purpose of this exercise is to help you learn to experience the presence of Jesus in a conversation with Him about a passage of scripture.
   c. You will also learn to journal, as you write down the impressions you have during your conversation with Him.

RECOVERING OUR LOST IDENTITY
MATURITY AND CAPACITY PART 1: WHAT IS MATURITY?

    d. This exercise is not intended to be a traditional Bible study or information gathering exercise that focuses on assimilating new information for the left hemisphere of your brain.

    e. Both hemispheres of the brain are involved as you read the scriptures, experience the presence of Jesus and interact with Him about the scriptures. This leads to spiritual formation and life transformation – not information accumulation.

3. Your facilitator will explain why there are scriptures on your worksheet.
    a. Notice the scripture from Genesis 4:18 on your worksheet. This scripture is listed because it is an example of a scripture that is not a very helpful passage to use for this exercise.
    b. The other scriptures listed on your worksheet are examples of scriptures that are easier to use for this exercise.

4. Your facilitator will review the following directions with you, and then demonstrate the exercise for you. To demonstrate this exercise, your facilitator will:
    a. Find a comfortable position.
    b. Choose a passage of scripture for the worksheet, and read it out loud.
    c. If any particular part of the passage catches his/her attention, your facilitator will stop and ask Jesus aloud what He would like him/her to know about or understand about it.
    d. If nothing in the passage catches his/her attention, your facilitator will wait until he/she has read the entire passage, and then ask Jesus what He would like him/her to know or understand about it. He/she can also ask the questions listed on the worksheet.
    e. Your facilitator will stop, listen and pay attention to any impression or thought that comes to mind. Your facilitator will report these impressions to you out loud and record them on the worksheet.
    f. Your facilitator will continue to dialogue with Jesus about the passage of scripture, ask questions, report impressions to you and write the impressions on the worksheet.
    g. Your facilitator will thank Jesus when the dialogue is complete.

5. Your facilitator will explain that because many of us perceive the presence of Jesus in different ways, this exercise emphasizes the "impressions" that we may experience during the exercise.
    a. Sometimes we become aware of new thoughts as we dialogue with Him.
    b. Sometimes, we may have a new picture in our mind that is based on the scripture or on our conversation with Jesus.
    c. Sometimes we may simply sense, feel and know that Jesus is with us.
    d. Focus your attention on perceiving His presence and experiencing His responses to you. Be open to Him making His presence known to you in creative and different ways. Record whatever impression of His presence you experience during the exercise.
    e. It is not necessary to record our experiences with phrases like, "Thus saith the Lord," or "God says."

6. Your facilitator will ask you to break into small groups of 3-5 people. When you have moved your chairs, please find a position that will be comfortable as you begin the exercise. You are welcome to remain in your seats, sit on the floor, lie down or stand up.

RECOVERING OUR LOST IDENTITY
MATURITY AND CAPACITY PART 1: WHAT IS MATURITY?

YOUR NOTES

7. Your facilitator will ask you to choose a passage of scripture from the worksheet. Your facilitator will give you the following instructions:
   a. Read the passage of scripture silently.
   b. If any particular part of the passage catches your attention, stop and silently ask Jesus what He would like you to know about or understand about it.
   c. If nothing in the passage catches your attention, wait until you have read the entire passage, and then silently ask Jesus what He would like you to know or understand about it. You can also ask the questions listed on the worksheet.
   d. Stop, listen and pay attention to any impression or thought that comes to your mind.
   e. Record your impression on your worksheet.
   f. Continue your conversation with Jesus about the passage of scripture, and record your impressions on your worksheet.
   g. When you have completed your dialogue, you may thank Jesus – or tell him what you appreciate about your time together.

8. When your facilitator has finished reading these instructions, you may begin your conversation with Jesus. You will have 5-10 minutes for this portion of the exercise. Your facilitator will help you by keeping track of time.

9. Your facilitator will let you know when it is time to begin sharing your impressions in your small group.
   a. Volunteers may take turns sharing their impressions from the exercise. Each person will have 3 minutes to share.
   b. Remember to stay relational by making eye contact as you share.
   c. When a group member is sharing, be supportive to them through active listening. It is not necessary to offer feedback, comments or criticism of their impressions.
   d. Your facilitator will help you by keeping track of time for you.

10. When small group sharing is finished, your facilitator may ask volunteers to share one or two words with the entire group that describe their experience with Jesus.

CLOSE THE GROUP WITH PRAYER

RECOVERING OUR LOST IDENTITY
MATURITY AND CAPACITY PART 1: WHAT IS MATURITY?

QUESTIONS FOR FURTHER DISCUSSION OR FOLLOW-UP

1. How do you define maturity? Why is maturity a lifetime journey?

2. What does it mean to you to be "fully alive like Christ?"

3. Why is your level of maturity not based on your physical age?

4. What do you think will happen to your individual and group identity as you mature?

5. Why do you need others to mature? Who are the people God has placed in your life to help you mature?

6. What is God's part in helping you mature? What is your part in developing your own maturity? Why is it important for you to know the difference?

7. Why do you need to learn to receive before you can give? Is it harder for you to receive than it is to give? Why?

8. Will you become more valuable as you become more mature? Why?

9. What are pseudo joy and pseudo maturity? Why do these give us the appearance of maturity?

10. Have BEEPS given you a sense of pseudo maturity? How did they do this? Be specific.

11. What happened to your pseudo maturity as stress increased? Be specific.

12. Explain this statement in your own words. "BEEPS are the result of a catastrophic failure to reach adult maturity – and keep us stuck in immaturity."

13. Why are Steps 10, 11 and 12 called "maintenance steps?" How can practicing these steps with a joyful and healing community help us grow and mature?

14. What did you experience in your conversation with Jesus about scripture in this week's exercise?

RECOVERING OUR LOST IDENTITY
MATURITY AND CAPACITY PART 1: WHAT IS MATURITY?

OPTIONAL 12-STEP QUESTIONS

1. Why is maturity an essential part of recovery?

2. Why are Steps 10, 11 and 12 called "maintenance steps?"

3. How can these steps help produce ongoing sobriety and maturity?

4. In your own words, what does Step 10 mean to you?

5. How can you continue to take your own inventory and promptly admit it when you are wrong? What people and resources do you need to help you?

6. What does Step 11 mean to you? Explain.

7. Do you know how to improve your conscious contact with God? Describe.

8. What did you experience in your conversation with Jesus about scripture in this week's exercise?

9. Can talking with Jesus about scripture help you improve your conscious contact with God? How?

10. Why is it important for you to pray for the knowledge of God's will for you, and the power to carry it out?

11. What does Step 12 mean to you?

12. What is a "spiritual awakening?" Have you had a spiritual awakening in recovery? How did this happen?

13. How can you carry the message of recovery to others who are attached to BEEPS? How can you do this now?

14. Would you like to practice Twelve Step and recovery principles in every part of your life? What does this practically mean for your life? Are there areas of your life in which you resist practicing these principles?

MY SCRIPTURE MEDITATION WORKSHEET

Don't choose a passage of scripture like this to learn this exercise:

> And unto Enoch was born Irad: and Irad begat Mehujael: and Mehujael begat Methusael: and Methusael begat Lamech. Genesis 4:18, KJV

Choose one of these passages of scripture for this exercise:

1. The Lord bless you and keep you; the Lord make his face shine upon you and be gracious to you. The Lord turn his face toward you and give you peace. Numbers 6:24-26, NIV

   Question: Why do You long to shine your face upon me?
   Why do You want me to know this?
   Why is there peace when Your face is toward me?

2. Keep your lives free from the love of money and be content with what you have, because God has said, "Never will I leave you; Never will I forsake you." So we say with confidence, "The Lord is my helper; I will not be afraid. What can man do to me?" Hebrews 13: 5-6, NIV

   Question: What does it mean that You will never leave me?
   Why don't I have to be afraid?

3. The Lord is my shepherd, I shall lack nothing. He makes me lie down in green pastures, he leads me beside quiet waters, He restores my soul. Psalm 23:1-3, NIV

   Question: Why do I lack nothing when You are with me?
   Where are the quiet waters?
   How do You want to restore my soul?

Record your impressions from this exercise here:

12 THE BLUEPRINT FOR A NEW YOU!
MATURITY AND CAPACITY PART 2: THE STAGES OF MATURITY

OPEN THE GROUP

- Ask for a volunteer to open the group in prayer.

EXERCISE: APPRECIATION AND MATURITY *10 Minutes*

Facilitator Note: Last week's lesson described maturity as a process of becoming more fully alive, in which we maximize our identity, reach our God-given potential, and use our gifts and skills wisely. These characteristics describe a person who is growing in maturity. It feels life giving to be in relationship with him or her.

In this exercise, participants will be asked to identify a person in their life who is maturing. Volunteers have the opportunity to share their appreciation for this person with their small group. This exercise helps review concepts of maturity from last week, and builds joyful capacity among participants. You can help participants complete this exercise by sharing your own appreciation and gratitude for a person who is maturing.

1. Break into small groups of 3-5 people.

2. Your facilitator will review some of the characteristics of maturity from last week's lesson. It feels life-giving to be with people who are maturing, because they are:
   a. Becoming more fully alive.
   b. Maximizing their unique identity.
   c. Reaching their God-given potential.
   d. Using gifts and skills wisely.

3. Your facilitator will share an appreciation moment about an experience he/she has had with a person in his/her own life who is maturing. While sharing, your facilitator will:
   a. Maintain eye contact.
   b. Identify the person and experience for which they are grateful.
   c. Describe the emotions they felt during the experience.
   d. Describe what their body felt like during the experience.

4. Your facilitator will ask volunteers to take turns sharing about their own experience with a person who is maturing. Each volunteer will have 2 minutes to share. Remember to:
   a. Maintain eye contact while sharing.
   b. Identify the person and experience for which you are grateful.
   c. Describe what emotions you felt during your experience.
   d. Describe what your body felt like during that experience.

5. Your facilitator will help you by keeping track of time.

6. When each group is finished, your facilitator may ask volunteers how they feel after the exercise with the entire group. Use one or two words to describe your feelings.

YOUR NOTES

THE BLUEPRINT FOR A NEW YOU!
MATURITY AND CAPACITY PART 2: THE STAGES OF MATURITY

YOUR NOTES

TODAY'S LESSON: Maturity and Capacity Part 2: The Stages of Maturity

> **Facilitator Note:** Play Session Twelve on the Restarting DVD.
> - Ask the class to follow along in their workbooks and take notes as needed.

CLASS NOTES: Maturity and Capacity Part 2: The Stages of Maturity

A quick review

Growth and maturity are god's ideas!
- Then God blessed them, and God said to them, "Be fruitful and multiply; fill the earth and subdue it..." Genesis 1: 28, NKJV

We are not born fully mature, physically or spiritually.

Maturity is a lifetime journey:
- Until we're all moving rhythmically and easily with each other, efficient and graceful in response to God's Son, fully mature adults, fully developed without and within, fully alive like Christ. Ephesians 4:11-13. The Message.

What are the stages of maturity?
- Where am I going?
- How will I know when I get there?

Maturity stages
- Unborn: pre-birth
- Infant: birth to 3 years old
- Child: age 4 to 12 years old
- Adult: age 13 to birth of first child
- Parent: until youngest child is 13
- Elder: begins when youngest child becomes an adult

The six stages of maturity consist of tasks and needs to be accomplished at each stage of life.

Unborn: pre-birth
- Grows a working body.

Infant: receives, learns, lives through joy
- Needs:
  - Joy bonds with both parents that are strong, loving, caring, secure
  - Important needs are met without asking
  - Quiet together time
  - Help regulating distress and emotions
  - Be seen through the "eyes of heaven"
  - Receive and give life
  - Have others synchronize with him/her first
- Tasks:
  - Receive with joy
  - Learn to synchronize with others
  - Organize self into a person through imitation
  - Learn to regulate emotions

THE BLUEPRINT FOR A NEW YOU!
MATURITY AND CAPACITY PART 2: THE STAGES OF MATURITY

- Learn to return to joy from every emotion
- Learn to be the same person over time
- Learn self-care skills
- Learn to rest

Child: develops an individual identity
- Needs:
  - Help to do what he or she does not feel like doing
  - Help sorting feelings, imaginations and reality
  - Feedback on guesses, attempts and failures
  - Be taught the family history
  - Be taught the history of God's family
  - Be taught the "big picture" of life
- Tasks:
  - Take care of self (one is enough for right now)
  - Learn to ask for what she or he needs
  - Self expression
  - Helping others understand you
  - Develop personal resources and talents
  - Learn to do "hard things"
  - Learn what satisfies
  - See self through the "eyes of heaven"

Adult: develops a group identity
- Needs
  - Time with peers to form a group identity
  - Inclusion in their same-gender community
  - Participation with same-gender leaders who use power fairly and well
  - Be given important tasks by their community
  - Feedback on their personal impact on history
  - Opportunities to share in life partnership
- Tasks
  - Take care of two or more at the same time
  - Discover the main characteristics of his heart
  - Bring self and others back to joy simultaneously
  - Develop a personal style that reflects her heart
  - Learn to protect others from himself or herself
  - Learn mutual satisfaction
  - Diversify and blend roles
  - Learn to express life-giving sexuality
  - Partnership

Young adults: the power years
- Power, relationships and truth are the three preoccupations of young adults.
- Particular attention must be given to their proper development during the "power years" of a young adult's life.

Young adults: power
- Observe adults using power wisely
- Do important tasks for her/his community
- Make an impact on history
- Learn significant roles
- Use sexual power wisely
- Protect others from himself/herself

THE BLUEPRINT FOR A NEW YOU!
MATURITY AND CAPACITY PART 2: THE STAGES OF MATURITY

Young adults: relationships
- Bond with peers
- Be included in the community of men/women
- Develop partnership relationships
- Achieve mutual satisfaction
- Bring self and others back to joy simultaneously

Young adults: truth
- Discover the main characteristics of her/his own heart
- Develop a personal style that reflects his/her heart
- Proclaim her/his true identity
  - Personal identity
  - Corporate identity
  - Spiritual identity

Parent: gives sacrificially to children
- Needs
  - To give life without requiring anything back
  - An encouraging partner
  - Guidance from elders
  - Peer review from other fathers or mothers
  - A secure and orderly environment
- Tasks
  - Building a home
  - Protecting his or her family
  - Serving his or her family
  - Enjoying his or her family
  - Maturing their children
  - Synchronizing with the developing needs of: spouse, children, family, work and church

Parent: singles
- Single people and spiritual parenting
- If you have matured appropriately you have a group identity, so:
  - Start with extended family
  - Focus on same gender
  - Have parenting coaches
  - Get peer support and review to determine when and if ready for spiritual parenting

Parent: spiritual parents
- God forms the family
- Your community affirms the call and relationship
- Your elders guide you
- 3 levels of spiritual adoption:
  - Supplemental: assist parents
  - Stand In: acting as parent for a time
  - Replacement: replaces one or both parents
    - Singles proceed with great caution
    - Infants need 2 bonds for life, gender issues, and needs of the infant

Elders: grow their community
- Needs
  - A community to call their own
  - Recognition by their community

THE BLUEPRINT FOR A NEW YOU!
MATURITY AND CAPACITY PART 2: THE STAGES OF MATURITY

- A proper place in the community structure
- Have others place trust in him or her
- Tasks
  - Hospitality
  - Giving life to the family-less
  - Being a "parent" for the community itself
  - Maintain their community's identity
  - Still act like him/herself in the midst of difficulty
  - Enjoy what God placed in each and everyone
  - Build the trust of others through the elder's own transparency and spontaneity

What are the perils of ignoring maturity?

The 4 level emotional control center in the right hemisphere of the brain
- Immaturity is pain at Level 3

The perils of ignoring maturity
- For though by this time you ought to be teachers, you need some one to teach you again the first principles of God's word. You need milk, not solid food; for every one who lives on milk is unskilled in the word of righteousness, for he is a child. But solid food is for the mature, for those who have their faculties trained by practice to distinguish good from evil. Hebrews 5:12-14, RSV

The perils of ignoring maturity
- Leadership failure
- Character weakness
- Emotional instability
- Fearful living
  - Marriage failures
  - Failure to thrive
  - BEEPS (addictions)

BEEPS
- There are many different types of BEEPS. Examples can include:
  - Behaviors: Work
  - Events: Thrill Seeking
  - Experiences: Sex
  - People: Relationships
  - Substances: Alcohol

BEEPS are a catastrophic failure to reach adult maturity – and block the development of further maturity.

Trauma A: the absence of necessary good things

Trauma B: bad things that happen

Steps to restoring maturity
- Check for wounds in your identity
- Identify your level of earned maturity
- Identify the "holes" in your maturity
- Identify the "next step"
- Identify community resources you need
- Pray for God to provide the resources
- Start to work

YOUR NOTES

THE BLUEPRINT FOR A NEW YOU!
MATURITY AND CAPACITY PART 2: THE STAGES OF MATURITY

The Twelve Steps are a relational program of recovery
- Relationship with God
  - Steps 1, 2, 3 and 11.
- Relationship with Self
  - Steps 4, 5, 6, 7 and 10.
- Relationship with Others
  - Steps 8, 9, and 12.
- Only when I work the Twelve Steps in a joyful, healing and maturing community can my maturity grow.

The "Thriving: Recover Your Life" training flow

Other modules in the Thriving: Recover Your Life training flow
- Belonging:
  - Thriving module for those who have completed Restarting or Forming
  - Helps build a joyful and thriving recovery community
  - Teaches the 19 skills the brain needs to thrive
- Forming:
  - Spiritual formation entrance to the Thriving training flow
  - Helps build a Christian character and identity that is joyful
- Healing
  - Designed for those who have completed Belonging
  - Continues the Immanuel Process that began in Restarting, Forming and Belonging
  - Helps participants experience the presence of God in a way that brings healing
  - Builds joyful and supportive healing community
- Loving
  - Designed for those who have completed the Healing module
  - Ongoing support for spiritual formation and recovery from trauma and BEEPS
  - Helps participants apply everything learned in other modules to relationships that are important to them
  - Following the completion of Loving, participants can identify relationships the would like to improve and repeat the entire Thriving process with those they love

EXERCISE: MATURITY ASSESSMENT *30 Minutes*

Facilitator Note: The purpose of this exercise is to help participants evaluate their progress in developing the skills that are essential for infant and child levels of maturity. In this self-assessment, participants focus on evaluating their progress on basic tasks that characterize these early and vital stages of maturity. To help you understand how to use this tool, please locate the maturity assessment, which is located in this chapter of your workbook. Please be sure to familiarize yourself with the assessment and these instructions before attempting to facilitate this exercise.

As you can see, the left side of the inventory contains the words "No, Sometimes, Usually and Always." These will allow participants to rate their level of progress in the development of specific tasks and traits of maturity. To the right, you will find a series of tasks highlighted in bold that are associated with first infant, and then child levels of maturity.

THE BLUEPRINT FOR A NEW YOU!
MATURITY AND CAPACITY PART 2: THE STAGES OF MATURITY

YOUR NOTES

There are 5 basic infant tasks and 6 basic child tasks listed on the inventory. Below each task are a series of statements that describe the specific traits that must be developed to master the task.

For example, under the infant stage of maturity, the first task is "The Infant Lives in Joy." Listed underneath "The Infant Lives in Joy," are the statements, "I am the same person over time" and "I know that I am seen through the 'eyes of heaven.'" Both of these statements describe traits that an infant must develop to live in joy.

To evaluate progress in the development of each maturity task, participants mark the "No, Sometimes, Usually or Always" box to the left of each trait. For example, in the case of the task "The Infant Lives in Joy," participants would mark the "No, Sometimes, Usually or Always" box to the left of the statements "I am the same person over time" and "I know that I am seen through the 'eyes of heaven.'" If a participant sometimes acts like the same person over time, they would mark the "Sometimes" box next to the statement "I am the same person over time." If they often see themselves through the eyes of heaven, they would mark the "Usually" box. An individual has mastered the infant level task of learning to "live in joy," if they typically are the same person over time, and know that they are seen through the eyes of heaven.

As participants complete this assessment for each infant and child maturity task, they will be able to recognize their level of maturity in these areas. This assessment covers only the infant and child levels of maturity, because individuals who are in early recovery from Trauma A, Trauma B and BEEPS tend to be stuck in an infant or in some cases, a child level of maturity.

It is important for participants to recognize several things as they complete their maturity assessment.

First, some people have great difficulty remembering their childhood, and many can't recall life before age 4. Without a memory of infancy or childhood, participants often wonder how they can complete the infant or child level assessments. For example, when assessing the infant task of "develops trust," participants may say, "I can't remember if quiet time together helped calm myself with people around'...I can't remember that far back.'" To help with this dilemma, it is useful to tell participants that the assessment is not asking them to remember their biological infancy or childhood. The assessment is asking them to determine whether they have skills associated with an infant or child level of maturity in the present. It is not asking them to evaluate their progress based on a partial or incomplete memory of the past.

For example, to assess the statement, "Quiet time together helped calm myself with people around," it is not necessary for a participant who is 40 years old to try to remember what was happening in their chronological infancy. They only need to determine whether they are able to share quiet time together and calm themselves with people around today at age 40. If, at age 40, they are unable to "share quiet time together and calm themselves," it is highly unlikely that they learned the skill before the age of 4. They would indicate "No" for the statement, "quiet time together helped calm myself with people around," regardless of their ability to remember their chronological infancy.

On the other hand, suppose that at age 40, they are usually able to quiet and calm themselves with people around. They can mark "Usually" next to the statement, "quiet time together helped calm myself with people around," regardless of their ability to remember their biological infancy. Even if they learned this skill when they were 39 years old, they

THE BLUEPRINT FOR A NEW YOU!
MATURITY AND CAPACITY PART 2: THE STAGES OF MATURITY

can still mark "Usually" next to the statement. The fact that they have some mastery of the skill – not the age at which they learned it – is what is important for the assessment. This assessment is asking participants to evaluate their progress based on their skill level today – and not based solely on partial or incomplete memory of the past.

Second, it is helpful to remind participants that the chronological ages associated with each stage indicate only the earliest possible ages in which we can reach and complete specific levels of maturity. Reaching a chronological age does not mean that we have reached a specific level of maturity. For example, the fact that a person is chronologically 27 years old does not necessarily mean that they have reached an adult level of maturity. Despite their age, they may remain stuck at an infant level of maturity if they have not completed the basic tasks associated with that level of earned maturity. It is entirely possible for a 27-year-old person to be stuck at an infant level of maturity – particularly if they have experienced significant Trauma A, Trauma B or have BEEPS attachments.

Third, be aware that the assessment does more than help evaluate our level of earned maturity. It also helps us recognize gaps or holes in maturity. Recognizing gaps or holes in maturity can help us identify the resources, people and community that are needed to help us grow in maturity. Becoming aware of these gaps helps us determine the "next step" in our journey to recovery and maturity.

How do gaps or holes in maturity occur? Gaps or holes in maturity happen when skills at a particular level of maturity are not adequately mastered. Even though many other skills consistent with that stage of maturity have been learned, gaps and holes can exist if there are other skills at that level that have been omitted – or are insufficiently developed.

For example, you will notice that one of the tasks that define an infant level of maturity is "Learns to Return to joy from every negative emotion." Suppose that an individual has mastered virtually all of the tasks needed to function at an infant level of maturity, and has learned to return to joy from every negative emotion except one – anger. Anger, as you may recall from week 3, is the emotion that drives us to "protect ourselves and make the pain stop." This inability to return to joy from anger is a gap or hole in maturity.

Practically speaking, this individual would be able to function at a higher level of maturity in almost every area of life – except when angry. When angry, this individual would return to an infant level of maturity, because they would be consumed with trying to protect themselves and make the pain stop – and would not be able to stay relational with others. This gap in maturity would repeatedly cause this person to revert – or fall back – into behaviors that are characteristic of an earlier level of maturity.

This gap will also sabotage attempts to work on some child level maturity tasks. For example, a skill associated with the development of a child level of maturity listed on the assessment is "Develops enough persistence to do hard things." Traits associated with that skill include "I can do hard things I don't feel like doing" and "I can control my cravings." The gap or hole in anger can significantly hurt this person's ability to master these child level tasks, because when angry, this person would be consumed with trying to protect themselves and make the pain stop. They would be unable to do hard things or control their cravings, because their entire focus would be on pain relief. The anger gap would lead to persistent difficulties associated with these child level tasks.

As participants complete their infant and child level assessments, it is helpful to encourage them to identify gaps in maturity. They should be aware that difficulties associated with tasks at a childhood level of maturity might be directly related to underlying gaps or holes that are present at the infant level. These gaps can't be fixed simply by working

THE BLUEPRINT FOR A NEW YOU!
MATURITY AND CAPACITY PART 2: THE STAGES OF MATURITY

harder at the child maturity tasks. They can only be resolved by recognizing the gap in maturity, and identifying the resources, people and community that are needed to fill in the gaps. This will help them accurately assess their problem and better understand the "next step" in building maturity. Work on developing the missing infant level maturity tasks can then begin!

Finally, please be aware that after completing their assessment, some participants may feel shame about their level of maturity. It can be hard for adults to recognize that they have spent most of their lives functioning at an infant or child level of maturity. For these reasons, it is important to emphasize the following:

- The assessment can help us celebrate and measure areas of growth. It is not intended to be a static, one time snapshot of maturity. By retaking the assessment over time, growth and maturity can be measured. Existing maturity – and growth in maturity can both be celebrated!
- The assessment is designed to help us identify areas in which we need to grow so that we can recognize the resources, community and people that we need to mature. Rather than being a negative experience, the assessment can empower us to move into the next phase of our recovery.
- The assessment is designed to help keep us safe. One of the surest ways to cause ourselves – and those around us – pain, is to take on responsibilities for things that we do not have the maturity to handle. By recognizing my level of maturity, I am able to assume responsibilities for tasks consistent with that level of maturity. I can avoid cycles of failure and pain by functioning within my level of earned maturity.
- This assessment helps me recognize and assume the growth and maturity tasks that provide the appropriate challenges that I need to grow. Recognizing the skills and traits needed for each level of maturity provides me a blueprint for growth that will help keep my growth focused.
- A small group sharing exercise in which volunteers are encouraged to share their results does not follow the assessment. This is a self-assessment exercise. Participants have the freedom to keep their results confidential.

As you lead participants through this exercise, please read each task and statement aloud. This will allow you to clarify any points to participants that are unclear as they complete their assessment.

YOUR NOTES

1. It is not necessary to break into small groups for the first part of this exercise.

2. Locate the maturity assessment in your workbook.

3. The purpose of this exercise is to help you assess your maturity and progress in developing the skills that are needed for infant and child levels of maturity. Listen as your facilitator explains:
   a. The assessment can help you celebrate and measure areas of growth. Over time, you will notice the growth of ongoing maturity.
   b. The assessment will help you answer the question, "What is my next step?" By helping you identify the areas in which you need to grow, you can begin to identify the resources, people and community that you need to mature.
   c. This assessment will help keep you safe. By recognizing your true level of maturity, you can avoid taking on responsibilities for which you do not have the maturity to handle.
   d. This assessment helps provide a blueprint for growth by identifying the tasks and challenges that are appropriate for your level of maturity.

THE BLUEPRINT FOR A NEW YOU!
MATURITY AND CAPACITY PART 2: THE STAGES OF MATURITY

    e. This assessment will help you identify gaps and holes in maturity that can keep you stuck and very frustrated. Gaps and holes in maturity can exist when we have not adequately mastered all of the skills needed at each level of maturity.
    f. This is a self-assessment exercise. You will not be asked to volunteer to share your assessment with anyone else.

4. Follow along on your assessment inventory as your facilitator explains how to complete the inventory.
   a. To the left side of the page are the words "No, Sometimes, Usually and Always." These help you describe the degree of progress you have made on specific maturity tasks.
   b. To the right, are a series of 5 basic infant tasks and 6 childhood tasks.
   c. The tasks are listed in bold.
   d. Below the tasks are a series of statements that describe the specific traits that must be developed to master the task.
   e. To complete the assessment, mark the "No, Sometimes, Usually or Always" box next to each statement.

5. Your facilitator will give you an example of how to complete the assessment.
   a. Find the task "Infant Lives in Joy" which is highlighted in bold on the first page of your assessment. It is the first task listed under the "Infant Stage" of maturity.
   b. Find the statements "I am the same person over time" and "I know I am seen through the 'eyes of heaven.'"
   c. Next to these statements are boxes for "No, Sometimes, Usually and Always."
   d. Simply mark either the "No, Sometimes, Usually or Always" box that most accurately describes the statements, "I am the same person over time" and ""I know I am seen through the 'eyes of heaven.'"
      i. If you are not the same person over time, mark the "No" box.
      ii. If you are sometimes the same person over time, mark the "Sometimes" box.
      iii. If you are usually the same person over time, mark the "Usually" box.
      iv. It you are always the same person over time, mark the "Always" box.
   e. You can complete the entire assessment in the same way.

6. This exercise is not asking you to base your answers solely on faulty or incomplete memories. It is asking you to determine whether you have the skills that are associated with an infant or child level of maturity in the present. Your facilitator will explain this example to you.
   a. Locate the second infant maturity task "develops trust" that is highlighted in bold. The statement "Quiet time together helped calm myself with people around" is one of the traits listed below it.
   b. If a person who is now 40 years old is unable to quiet and calm themselves with people around, it is unlikely that they learned this in biological infancy. They would mark the "No" box next to this statement, even if they can't remember their biological infancy.
   c. If a person is now 40 years old, and usually is able to quiet and calm themselves with people around, they would mark the "Usually" box. They would mark the "Usually" box even if they can't remember learning this skill as a biological infant.
   d. If a person is now 40 years old and learned this skill "Sometimes" at age 39, they would mark the "Sometimes" box, even if they can't remember their biological infancy.
   e. The emphasis is on identifying skills that we have in the present – not trying to remember the distant past.

7. The ages listed on the assessment represent the earliest that it is possible for you

THE BLUEPRINT FOR A NEW YOU!
MATURITY AND CAPACITY PART 2: THE STAGES OF MATURITY

YOUR NOTES

to have developed all of the skills associated with a specific level of maturity. Your facilitator will explain:
   a. Reaching a certain biological age does not mean that we have developed a corresponding level of maturity.
   b. For example, a person may be 27 years old, but stuck at an infant level of maturity.
   c. They may remain stuck at that level of maturity until they are able to develop the skills and learn the tasks associated with that level of maturity.
   d. It is likely that a person who has experienced significant Trauma A, Trauma B and/or attachments to BEEPS may be stuck at an infant or child level of maturity.

8. This assessment helps you identify gaps or holes in maturity. Gaps or holes in maturity may happen when skills at a particular level of maturity are not adequately mastered. Even if other skills in that level of maturity are learned, gaps in maturity may remain if other skills at that level have been omitted – or insufficiently developed. Your facilitator will explain this example of a gap relating to anger at a childhood level of maturity:
   a. Find the infant skill, "Learns to return to joy from every negative emotion." Under it, you will see a list of the big six negative emotions. To develop an infant level of maturity, it is necessary to learn to return to joy from every negative emotion, including anger.
   b. If a person has not learned to return to joy from anger, but has learned every other infant level maturity task, they will have a gap in maturity associated with anger.
   c. They would function at a higher level of maturity in every area of life – except when they are angry. Their inability to return to joy from anger means that they would revert to an infant level of maturity when they are angry. They would be consumed with trying to protect themselves and make the pain stop – and would not be able to stay connected relationally to others when they are angry.
   d. The anger gap in maturity will also tend to sabotage efforts to develop skills at a child level of maturity. On your worksheet, locate the third child maturity task which is, "Develops enough persistence to do hard things." Below it are the traits, "I can do hard things I don't feel like doing" and "I can control my cravings."
   e. Being able to return to joy from anger is a prerequisite for developing these traits of childhood maturity. If I am unable to return to joy from anger, I will be unable to do hard things and control my cravings when I'm angry, because I'll be consumed with trying to protect myself and make my pain stop.
   f. This difficulty associated with childhood maturity tasks can only be resolved by addressing the underlying gaps at the infant level of maturity. Recognizing the gaps helps me get "unstuck," and identify the resources, community and people I need to mature.

9. Your facilitator will help you begin the assessment.
   a. Your facilitator will read each task and statement aloud, and will answer any questions that you may have.
   b. Reflect on each statement, and mark "No, Sometimes, Usually or Always" next to each statement.

10. When you have completed the assessment, your facilitator will remind you that:
    a. You do not have to share your assessment with anyone.
    b. You can use your assessment to identify the gaps, and identify the resources, community and people that you need to mature.
    c. You can celebrate your progress, and return to the assessment again in the future as you mature.

CLOSE THE GROUP WITH PRAYER

MY MATURITY ASSESSMENT WORKSHEET

Follow your facilitator's instructions as you complete your worksheet.

No	Sometimes	Usually	Always	
				Infant stage: Ideal age: birth through age 4
				1. The infant lives in joy. The infant learns to expand their capacity for joy.
				The Infant also learns that joy is one's normal state and builds joy strength.
				a. I am the same person over time
				b. I know I am seen through the "eyes of heaven"
				2. Develops trust
				a. I have experienced strong loving bonds with mother or another woman.
				b. I have experienced strong loving bonds with father or another man.
				c. Important needs were met until I learned to ask.
				d. Quiet time together helped calm myself with people around.
				e. Others took the lead and synchronized with me and my feelings first.
				3. Learns how to receive
				a. I receive with joy and without guilt or shame.
				4. Begins to organize self into a person through relationship
				a. I know how to rest and quiet myself.
				b. I can receive and give life.
				c. I can now synchronize with others and their feelings.
				d. I found people to imitate so now I have a personality I like.
				5. Learns how to return to joy from every unpleasant emotion
				a. I learned how to regulate and quiet the big "six" emotions:
				1. Anger
				2. Fear
				3. Sadness
				4. Disgust
				5. Shame
				6. Hopelessness/Despair
				b. I can return to joy from every emotion and restore broken relationships
				1. Anger
				2. Fear
				3. Sadness
				4. Disgust
				5. Shame
				6. Hopelessness/Despair

MY MATURITY ASSESSMENT WORKSHEET

No	Sometimes	Usually	Always	
				Child Stage: Ideal age 4 through 12
				1. The child can ask for what is needed – can say what one thinks or feels
				a. I can ask for what I need.
				b. I enjoy self-expression.
				2. Learns what brings personal satisfaction
				a. I know what satisfies me.
				b. I can take care of myself.
				3. Develops enough persistence to do hard things
				a. I can do hard things I don't feel like doing.
				b. I can do hard things (even if they cause me some pain.)
				c. I am comfortable with reasonable risks, attempts and failures.
				d. I can control my cravings.
				4. Develop personal resources and talents
				a. I am growing in the things I am good at doing (my personal resources and talents)
				b. I have received love – I don't have to earn it.
				c. I can see myself through the "eyes of heaven".
				5. Knows self and takes responsibility to make self understood to others
				a. I help other people to understand me better if they don't respond well to me
				b. I can separate my feelings, my imagination and reality in my relationships
				6. Understand how she/he fits into history as well as "Big Picture" of what life is about
				a. I know how my family came to be the way it is in family history.
				b. I know how God's family came to be the way it is.
				c. I know the "Big Picture" of life with the stages of maturity.

RESTARTING
FACILITATOR NOTES

RESTARTING
FACILITATOR RESOURCES

GETTING STARTED

Now that you are interested in developing and facilitating a Restarting group, the following steps will help you learn to use the Restarting materials to move forward.

Before you buy a Facilitator Package or the Restarting DVDs
Please visit our website at www.thrivingrecovery.org or watch the Restarting promotional video. This video provides an overview of the Restarting module, and includes previews of weekly lessons from the Restarting DVDs. You can sample Restarting before making a decision to purchase Restarting DVDs or the facilitator package.

Determine the setting in which you will be using Restarting
It is important that you determine the setting in which you will develop a Restarting group, because there are three different licensed versions of the Restarting DVD series. Only two licenses permit group use. Select either an *Open Group License* or an *Institutional/Training License* if you plan to facilitate a Restarting group. Please be sure that you order the series that is most appropriate for your setting. The three series and licenses are:

OPEN GROUP LICENSE
Under the Open Group License, individuals, churches or community groups can use the Restarting videos, name and materials as long as they do not profit materially or financially from its use. Under the Open Group License, organizations and individuals may request donations or have participants share expenses for this license and materials. Any use of this material in commercial or training venues where admission, enrollment, participation or tuition is charged is prohibited under the Open Group License.

The Open Group License Restarting materials package is designed to help you develop and begin a new Restarting group. This package includes: (Exact contents subject to change.)
- The Restarting DVD series, containing all 12 Restarting lessons
- The Restarting facilitator's DVD
- The "Banana Baseball" DVD
- Four Restarting workbooks
- A short Restarting promotional video
- 50 Restarting brochures
- A Thriving meeting banner

The images in the Open Group DVD Series are included on 4 DVDs, and the image quality is excellent for use on larger screens in a group setting. Available from Shepherd's House Inc. www.lifemodel.org or www.thrivingrecovery.org.

INSTITUTIONAL/TRAINING USE
Purchase of the Institutional/Training Restarting License is required when participants are charged an admission, enrollment, tuition or other participation fees for Restarting or when Restarting groups are conducted as part of such a program. Institutional use of Restarting materials by both for-profit and not-for profit organizations requires a separate, current Institutional/Training License from Shepherd's House Inc.

The images in the Institutional/Training Video Series are included on 12 DVDs. The image compression on the Institutional/Training DVDs makes these images superior to either the Home Use or Open Group DVDs. Because there is only one lesson per DVD the disks can be used for multiple classes simultaneously. Available from Shepherd's House Inc. www.lifemodel.org or www.thrivingrecovery.org.

RESTARTING
FACILITATOR RESOURCES

HOME USE

Purchasers of the Restarting video series Home Use License may use the video for their own personal and private use only. The Home Use License does not permit use of the video in groups, classes, training or where the licensee may profit materially or financially from its use.

The Home Use DVD Series is designed for personal study and review. Because the Home Use DVD series costs substantially less than the other DVD series licenses, it is a good choice for anyone wishing to view the entire Restarting video series before purchasing the Open Group License or the Institutional/Training License needed to lead Restarting groups. The images on the Home Use DVD series are excellent for use at home, and have been edited and compressed so that the entire series fits on only 2 DVDs.

USING MY RESTARTING DVD SERIES, WORKBOOK AND FACILITATOR MATERIALS.

The following steps will help you learn to use the facilitator materials, and navigate through the process of developing your Restarting group.

Check for updates on the facilitator's page of the Thriving Recovery website
The facilitator's page on the Thriving Recovery website will have the latest facilitator training updates, notes and announcements. In addition, all scheduled facilitator training retreats will be posted there. Visit www.thrivingrecovery.org for details.

Watch the Restarting DVD series and read your workbook thoroughly
You need to understand the flow and content of Restarting before you attempt to facilitate a Restarting group. Read the Restarting workbook and fill in the answers to all questions. It will be helpful to complete the "Questions for Further Discussion or Follow-up," that follow each group session since these can serve as a Restarting study guide for facilitators as well as for groups. Reading the detailed facilitator notes and step-by-step instructions will help you learn to lead each Restarting exercise.

Watch the Facilitator Video
The Restarting facilitator video contains instructions, demonstrations and examples for all the inner healing and brain training exercises in each Restarting session. The Facilitator video also includes information that will help explain the "Facilitator Notes" section of your workbook, as well as a presentation entitled the "Future of Recovery."

Watch the "Banana Baseball" video by Jim Wilder
Banana Baseball will give you an overview of science and theory behind the Thriving Recover Your Life programs that include Restarting. Jim Wilder created this video to introduce the concepts of brain science and spirituality as they apply to addiction and recovery. In this video, Jim describes addiction as a "catastrophic failure to reach adult maturity." He presents the brain science behind the development of addiction, and how addictions can be used to "turn off" internal pain and distress.

Determine if you will attend a facilitator training retreat
As mentioned previously, the best way to prepare to facilitate a Restarting group is by attending a 2-3 day Restarting facilitator training retreat. These training retreats provide you with relational training that will help you – and your new group Thrive! Please check the Thriving Recovery website for training dates and locations – or to schedule a facilitator training retreat at your location.

Meet with your pastor or supervisor/program director
It is vital that you meet with your pastor or supervisor/program director before beginning, or announcing your intention to begin, a Restarting group. His or her permission and support is vital to the development, success and integration of your group within existing ministry or program structures. Without proper preparation the Belonging group that follows Restarting will have little chance of success. Part of the hope provided by the Thriving: Recover Your Life program rests on a new relationship between recovery groups and their communities in order to achieve a higher level of successful recoveries. Setting up the program correctly is vital to your success.

RESTARTING
FACILITATOR RESOURCES

In your meeting it will be important to explain your desire, purpose and strategy for developing a Restarting group. Your pastor or supervisor should also understand the entire Thriving training flow. Explain the steps and preparations you have made to facilitate the group. You should make sure that you allow enough time to review this Restarting workbook and facilitator guide, the Restarting DVD Series and the Restarting promotional video.

It is also a good idea to:
- Discuss strategy for publicizing and announcing the new group. The Restarting promotional DVD is an excellent tool to introduce Restarting to churches, ministries and programs.
- Discuss the formation and development of the Restarting facilitator leadership team.
- Explain that it is not a good idea to establish a Thriving crisis group until a core of participants have experienced Restarting and can respond appropriately to those in acute crisis. Restarting is not intended to provide the level of intervention and assistance needed for those in severe crisis. It is recommended that those working in the crisis group have completed all available Thriving modules before attempting to facilitate a crisis group.

DEVELOP YOUR RESTARTING FACILITATOR TEAM

After receiving permission and creating a leadership plan for a Restarting group, invite your leadership team to view the Restarting DVD series. Team members should read this entire Restarting workbook and facilitator guide. View the facilitator video together. Practice the exercises as a group. Build some joy together!

Use your Restarting promotional video and publicize the start of your group
The Restarting promotional video is designed for use in churches, ministries and other organizations, to provide an introduction to Restarting and the entire Thriving program. It can be used during a community meeting, staff meeting or training session – or in a Sunday morning service. Be creative in announcing the beginning of Restarting. Joy is contagious!

Use your Restarting brochures
Designate the contact person from your Restarting facilitator team, and place their contact information and Restarting meeting location on the back of your brochures. Brochures help you contact individuals, groups and agencies who may not be familiar with Thriving Recovery or Restarting.

Post your group on the Life Model discussion group forum
Please visit www.lifemodel.org. You will be able to post the location and meeting time for your group on that website. Check for forums that may develop on www.thrivingrecovery.org as well.

Hang your restarting banner and meet
The Restarting banner that is included in your facilitator materials can be displayed as appropriate to mark the location of the Restarting meeting room or building so that participants can find it easily.

FACILITATOR TRAINING

Why do I need training to facilitate a Restarting group?
As you read this workbook, you will discover that Restarting is very different from most other approaches to recovery from trauma, addiction and painful character growth issues. Over 30 brain training and inner healing exercises are contained in this workbook that require a different set of facilitator skills and training from other recovery groups. At the heart of each Restarting session are joy and relationship building exercises that help our brains heal and overcome the devastating effects of trauma, pain and addiction. Inner healing exercises help us learn to experience the presence of Jesus. These should be common experiences but they are not.

RESTARTING
FACILITATOR RESOURCES

While your workbook contains detailed facilitator notes and step-by-step instructions to help you lead each exercise, you will discover that the best way to learn the exercises is to experience them personally. Personal experience and training, combined with the notes and instructions located in the workbook, will provide you with the best preparation to facilitate a Restarting group. For this reason, you are strongly encouraged to participate in Restarting facilitator training prior to beginning a Restarting group. Please consider each of the following training resources.

The Restarting facilitator training video
The Restarting facilitator training video explains and demonstrates of each Restarting exercises. This invaluable training resource helps you learn and review each exercise. The combination of the facilitator training video with the notes and instructions in this Restarting workbook and facilitator's guide will help prepare you to lead your group.

The Thriving Recovery website
The Thriving Recovery website (www.thrivingrecovery.org) will contain the most updated postings about Restarting training. To provide you with the best training experience and materials possible, Restarting facilitator training will continue growing over time. As facilitator training grows and develops, new training ideas, insights and materials will be posted.

Participate in a Restarting group
One of the best ways you can prepare to facilitate a Restarting group is by participating in a Restarting group in your area. This will allow you to learn, practice and experience a weekly Restarting group before attempting to facilitate your own group. After you have completed 12 weeks of Restarting, you will be better prepared to attend a Restarting facilitator retreat. Please check the Thriving Recovery website for the location of a Restarting group near you.

Attend a Restarting facilitator retreat
The best way to prepare to facilitate a Restarting group is by attending a 2-3 day Restarting facilitator training retreat. Be sure that you have read your workbook and watched each Restarting DVD before you attend. This short, but intensive, training experience will help you:
- Learn and practice each Restarting exercise with other Restarting facilitators.
- Experience a sample Restarting session.
- Better understand the flow and overview of Restarting and the entire Thriving program.
- Hear foundational presentations about the future of recovery, training and leadership.
- Network with other Restarting facilitators.
- Ask questions that will help you learn and apply Restarting material and exercises.

To find out more about Restarting facilitator retreats, please visit www.thrivingrecovery.org. Scheduled training dates and locations will be posted here. The website will also help you find out how to request a Restarting facilitator retreat in your area.

RESTARTING
FACILITATOR RESOURCES

FACILITATOR NOTES

As you begin your journey through recovery with your group, I want you to know how much your gift of leadership is appreciated. The gifts of your heart, joy, hard-earned maturity, and ongoing recovery from the pain of trauma, addictions and character growth issues are priceless. These gifts, combined with your faithfulness, hard work and prayers can empower you – and your group – to become a healing community that empowers recovery, and helps people begin to rebuild lives that have been devastated by the pain of trauma, addictions and character growth issues.

We each long for a destiny that is greater than the sum of our problems. We don't just want to recover from our problems – we want to be made fully alive. We want our recovery, lives and relationships – everything about us – to Thrive. By facilitating your Restarting group, you are offering participants the opportunity to begin their recovery – and walk more fully into the unique destiny and life that God has created for them.

WHAT IS RESTARTING?
Restarting is the first module in the Thriving: Recover Your Life series. It is the "recovery" entrance into the Thriving program, because it is designed to help participants begin – or restart – their recovery from trauma, addictions, or other character growth issues. As you will discover, Restarting is a revolutionary approach to the problems of trauma and addictions. Over the next 12 weeks, you and your group will experience the following Restarting lessons:
- Train Your Brain for Change!
- The 2 Skills Your Brain Can't Live Without
- Calming Our Painful Emotions.
- Strategies That Keep You Stuck
- Healthy Relationships
- Painful Relationships
- Toxic Relationships
- Trauma, Hope and Recovery
- Leaving Codependency Behind
- Attachments That Kill: How Addictions Re-wire Your Brain
- Recovering Our Lost Identity
- The Blueprint For A New You

Restarting is much more than a recovery program that is based on learning new information. Information does not usually lead to change – and this is especially true in recovery from the pain of trauma and addictions. Restarting is different, because it consists primarily of joy, relationship building and inner healing exercises that help you and your brain heal from trauma and addictions.

HOW IS EACH RESTARTING LESSON ORGANIZED?
Each Restarting lesson has three basic components. Because Restarting is a solution-centered approach to recovery, our emphasis is primarily on helping participants learn and develop new joy and relationship-building skills that help change the brain. As a result, only about 1/3 of each Restarting session is devoted to teaching, and approximately 2/3 of our time is spent on joyful brain training and inner healing exercises.

Teaching
The teaching portion of each week's Restarting lesson is on DVD. Teaching notes for each lesson are listed in the corresponding chapter of the workbook. Each week's lesson is progressive, and builds on the foundation of material learned in previous weeks. The lessons also contain a review of material from previous weeks, so that new members or those who missed a week will be able to catch up. A more detailed overview of each chapter may be found in the Facilitator Chapter Overview section of your workbook. You do not have to teach this material to lead a Restarting group!

Brain training – and joy and relationship building exercises
Facilitator notes and step-by-step instructions for each exercise are located in every chapter of the workbook. Each exercise is designed to help participants build joy and learn new relationship skills together. These exercises help build new brain skills that are needed for recovery and the development of ongoing maturity.

RESTARTING
FACILITATOR RESOURCES

Inner healing
The inner healing portion of Restarting lessons consists of a powerful combination of video and exercises that help participants learn to experience the presence of Jesus. The videos are included as part of the weekly teaching sessions on DVD, and facilitator notes and step-by-step instructions for exercises that help participants learn to experience the presence of Jesus are located in the workbook.

What is included in the weekly Restarting DVD lessons?
The weekly DVD Lessons provides facilitators and participants with the following:
- A standard introduction and overview of the Thriving: Recover Your Life program.
- An introduction to this week's topic.
- This week's 3 dimensional living brain moment.
- Scriptural principles that provide a foundation for the lesson.
- A focus on essential aspects of brain training – and the emotional control center, which is located in the right hemisphere of the brain.
- Attachments to BEEPS – and recovery.
- This week's 12 Step principle.
- Instructions for facilitators to turn off and restart the video so that the group can practice exercises based on the lesson, when needed.
- Four of the weekly lessons conclude with video of live inner healing sessions from Dr. Karl Lehman.

As the DVD plays, participants can follow along with teaching notes contained in their workbook. To make it easier for participants, all text seen on the DVD is listed in the teaching notes.

What is included in each chapter of the Restarting workbook?
Each chapter of the workbook contains teaching notes from the DVD. Please be aware that a facilitator's overview and guide to each chapter is located in the Facilitator's Chapter Overview section in the back of the workbook. In addition, each chapter contains important information for both facilitators and participants, including:
- A reminder to begin each group in prayer.
- Weekly in-group exercises that help build joy and improve brain training.
- In-depth facilitator notes and step-by-step instructions that help you lead each Restarting exercise, including the time allotted for each.
- Teaching notes that contain all the text displayed on the screen during the week's DVD lesson.
- Questions for further study that can be used for homework or for a separate discussion group.
- A second set of questions based on the 12 Steps that can be used in a separate discussion group.
- Optional exercises if needed.
- Worksheets needed for in-group exercises.

What do I need to facilitate a Restarting group?
As the group facilitator, you will need the Restarting DVD set, which contains the teaching segment of each week's lesson. In addition, you and each member of your leadership team will need a Restarting workbook. I strongly recommend that you make every effort to watch each DVD lesson in advance. To lead the group, you are also going to have to review the facilitator notes and prepare for each week's exercises ahead of time. You will also need to read the chapter overview contained in the Facilitator's Chapter Overview section of the workbook.

Participants will also need their own copy of the Restarting workbook. As you have seen, each chapter of the workbook contains teaching notes, exercise instructions, worksheets and questions for further study. Without the workbook, participants will feel very frustrated, because they won't be able to keep up with the information presented on the DVD, and they won't have the other materials in each chapter that are needed for group work. Whether you provide workbooks for participants, or ask them to pre-order their workbooks prior to the first Restarting session, you will need to make sure that each member has one before group begins.

In addition to the DVD and workbooks you will need the following equipment to facilitate a Restarting group:
- DVD player.
- A TV that is big enough for all participants to see easily.
- Extension cords or power strips as needed.

RESTARTING
FACILITATOR RESOURCES

- A microphone or sound amplification equipment – if needed – so that everyone in the room can hear you easily.
- Equipment to play music or audio files if you choose to use optional exercises included in some chapters.

What kind of meeting place do I need?
Restarting is intended to be highly flexible so that it can be used in a variety of settings and locations. Restarting groups can meet in churches, schools, homes, the workplace, residential or outpatient recovery or halfway house programs, jails, prisons, youth programs, crisis pregnancy programs, training centers – or wherever it is needed.

Regardless of where your group is located, you will need to choose a room that you can use regularly for the entire 12 week module. The room should have a door that closes and be free of outside distractions. If possible, choose a room with a good source of light. Since some participants may want to sit or lie down on the floor during relaxation exercises, having a carpet or floor covering will be helpful.

The size of the room will depend on the size of your group. Please be aware that some of the exercises will require your group to get up and walk around in groups – so choose a room that gives everyone a good bit of breathing space. Your room will also have to be large so that participants can easily re-arrange their chairs for the weekly small group exercises.

You should also pay attention to the physical layout of your room. To begin with, you will need to make sure that you place the TV where everyone can see it. You will also need to make sure that a TV and DVD player are available in the room – or bring them with you. Please also pay attention to the location of electrical outlets, and bring extension cords or power strips if needed. If you need help setting up or using any of this equipment, be sure to ask for help before your group starts.

To set up chairs, it is helpful to arrange them in rows facing you and the TV. Depending on the physical size and dimensions of your room, arranging the chairs in rows may make it easier for all to watch the DVD. If you prefer, you may also set up chairs in circular rows, and if you do so, make sure that you leave the top of the circle open for you and the TV. Please be aware that there is always an introductory Restarting exercise before the DVD lesson. This means that in some weeks, participants will have to move their chairs to form small groups – and then back again before watching the video.

What are the ground rules that can help keep my group safe?
Keeping your group safe is one of your most important tasks as a facilitator. Please make sure that all participants are aware of the following ground rules for Restarting:
- Confidentiality is a fundamental group rule. Confidentiality means that what an individual participant in a Restarting group shares should never be repeated by another participant outside of group at any time – without explicit permission in advance. Participants should also know that facilitators may have a legal obligation to report anything shared that indicates:
  - A person is in immediate danger of hurting themselves, others or the property of others.
  - Child abuse or abuse of the elderly.
- Exercises that help participants build joyful bonds together are powerful. For this reason, all small group exercises must be done in groups of 3-5 people. The only possible exceptions to this ground rule are in the cases of a married couple – or parent and child, and these should be approved by you in advance. Personal "couple bonds" between 2 unmarried persons should be discouraged.
- Participation in all group exercises is encouraged – but voluntary.
- Feedback offered in small group exercises should be consistent with the instructions given with that exercise.
- Since all group exercises are designed to help build joy and brain skills, group interactions should be supportive. Personal advice and criticism are never appropriate.
- Restarting participants should arrive for group without being intoxicated or under the influence of psychoactive drugs Intoxication or the use of mind-altering BEEPS keeps the brain from being able to learn and train. A brain that is not sober is a brain that is not able to learn or train! If a participant is under the influence, they may be referred to a Thriving crisis group (if available) or invited to return the following week when sober.
- Threats, intimidation or violence of any kind will result in immediate dismissal from group.

As a facilitator, it is your job to help make sure that your group remains safe by following these simple ground rules. If these ground rules are broken, it is helpful to keep these things in mind.
- Stay relational with the person who has broken a group ground rule. By staying relational, you maintain a personal connection that will help them return to joy from the shame they may experience.

RESTARTING
FACILITATOR RESOURCES

- In almost all cases, you will only need to remind a participant of a particular ground rule. A simple reminder is enough to help them change their behavior.
- If repeated reminders are not enough to help participants observe the ground rules, you may need to take other actions. These may include:
  - Asking them to stay home and miss group for a week.
  - Referring them to the Thriving crisis group.
  - Ask them not to return to Restarting.
- A Violation of a participant's confidentiality is very serious. Few things will destroy a group faster than gossip. For this reason, depending on the nature and severity of the violation, you may need to:
  - Ask them to stay home and miss group for a week.
  - Refer them to the Thriving crisis group (if available.)
  - Ask them not to return to Restarting until you have met with them and the issue is resolved.
- Violence, threats or intimidation are never acceptable. In these cases, you will likely need to:
  - Immediately ask the participant to leave group and go home for the evening.
  - Ask them not to return to Restarting for a minimum of 12 weeks.
  - If appropriate, they may attend the crisis group (if available.)
  - Meet with them prior to any future participation in Restarting.

What else do I need to know that will help me facilitate Restarting?
- Restarting is not just for your group – it is for you too! Helping people begin their journey into recovery and destiny is an amazing task, but it's even better when you are growing more fully alive in the process. This means that it is important for you to continue your own recovery, and build joyful, secure and life giving relationships with others as you lead your group. Do not neglect your own growth!

- It is helpful if you have your own personal support team. To be successful, you are going to need your own network of supportive and empowering relationships with others – and God – that will help you maintain your own joyful capacity. You are also going to need ongoing prayer support during this process.

- It is a very good idea to adopt a team leadership approach to Restarting. Team leadership has several important implications.
  - Having a team of leaders in your group means that you will have ongoing support during group.
  - Team members can build joy together – and this helps keep your leadership healthy.
  - Team members can be an extra set of eyes that can help spot members who are confused or who need extra help to complete an exercise.
  - A team approach to leadership means that your group will be able to maintain continuity if one member of the team is sick, or has to miss a Restarting session.
  - It is a good idea to designate a primary leader for the entire Restarting module. While other team members may help facilitate specific exercises, having a primary leader establishes continuity, which helps the group feel safer and more comfortable.
  - It is also a good idea for a leadership team to have at least one member who is receiving "on the job training" to facilitate the next Restarting group.

- Preparing in advance for each Restarting lesson is very important. Be sure to read each chapter and prepare to lead each exercise ahead of time. It is also helpful to watch the weekly Restarting video and facilitator's video before each session. Pay close attention to the facilitator notes and step-by-step instructions that accompany each Restarting exercise. You will have to prepare for each of these exercises in advance, and demonstrate them for participants.

- Please keep in mind that all Restarting exercises are designed for groups of 3-5 people. Exercises that build joyful bonds are powerful. Practicing our joy and relationship building skills in groups of 3-5 people helps keep participants safer as their lives are Restarting. It is a good idea to remind participants of this ground rule weekly.

- BEEPS is an important Restarting concept that you should know from the beginning. In Restarting lessons, we very rarely use the term "addictions." Instead, we use the term "BEEPS," which stands for Behaviors, Events, Experiences, People or Substances that help the brain artificially medicate pain that it is unable to regulate internally. The concept of BEEPS is very useful for describing the problem of addictions – and it also helps participants understand and

RESTARTING
FACILITATOR RESOURCES

develop the brain skills they need to overcome and displace the need for these harmful attachments.

- As you plan your Restarting group, pay attention to the optional exercises at the end of each chapter of the workbook. One set of questions is based on the weekly DVD lesson and workbook exercises and the other set focuses on helping participants apply the 12 Steps to Restarting concepts. These questions can be used privately by participants to further their own growth, or they can be used to develop weekly discussion groups that meet at other times during the week. Since participation in a joyful and supportive community is essential for recovery, these discussion groups could help provide another point of contact for group members. Should you choose to hold one or two weekly discussion groups, be sure that participants understand that the discussion groups are supplements to – and not replacements for the main weekly Restarting lesson.

- Restarting is designed to allow new members to join at any time. It is not a closed group. For this reason, review is built into each lesson, and Participants are also encouraged to repeat Restarting until they have completed every chapter in their workbook.

- Start your group on time. Each Restarting lesson is designed to last for 90 minutes. If you start your group late, you will not have enough time to complete the weekly exercises listed in the workbook. You may choose to schedule your group for 2 hours if you would like to give your group extra time for the exercises and discussion.

- Restarting is not intended to build "couple bonds" between two people who are not married. When joy is built, attachments can grow – and this is why all Restarting exercises must be done in groups of 3-5 people. The development of "couple bonds" is entirely discouraged between two people of the same sex – or opposite sex. Should you become aware of two participants who are developing these bonds, it is a good idea to discuss the issue with them. The outcome of relationships between two people who are wounded and in need of recovery is usually negative – and usually leads to BEEPS and relapse.

1 TRAIN YOUR BRAIN FOR A CHANGE
HOW IS THE BRAIN ORGANIZED? WHAT DOES IT NEED?

FACILITATOR NOTES

This introductory lesson is the first in a four week series, and helps participants understand how the brain is organized and trained. Foundational research that describes how the brain is organized, developed and trained opens new frontiers for recovery from trauma, addictions and character growth issues. New solution-based approaches that help re-train the brain are possible.

How the brain is organized and what it needs for training are the subjects of this week's lesson. The lesson begins with a discussion of the function of the two hemispheres of the brain, and introduces the significance of the emotional control center in the right hemisphere of the brain. Participants learn that the brain and emotional control center are organized, developed and trained in our first year of life through non-verbal interactions with others. These first-year, non-verbal interactions form the basis of our ability to regulate emotions for the rest of our lives.

Our emotional control center, and entire brain, develops best when we are in relationship with others who are joyful. Non-verbal, eye-to-eye interactions with others who are empowered by joy teach the brain to regulate emotions, and form the basis for the development of the entire brain. These interactions literally train our brain to regulate the neurotransmitter dopamine effectively. In addition to playing a crucial role in the brain's growth and development, dopamine also helps us to feel pleasure. When we are able to internally regulate dopamine effectively, joy becomes our natural state.

As we experience ongoing, non-verbal, eye-to-eye communication with others who are empowered by joy, our own capacity for joy increases. Our growing joy strength allows us to handle the pain and stress of life without being overwhelmed. Building ever-increasing capacity for joy is a task for the first year of life.

When we don't regulate dopamine effectively, our joyful capacity is low and we are frequently unable to live in joy. Our level of pain tends to overwhelm our level of joy, and this experience is traumatic. In response, the brain embarks on a quest to find something that will artificially regulate dopamine, increase joy, and eliminate distress. The brain will tend to develop attachments to BEEPS (Behaviors, Events, Experiences, People or Substances) that can artificially regulate dopamine, emotions, pleasure and pain. BEEPS medicate emotions and pain that the brain can't regulate internally.

Because these attachments to BEEPS help regulate dopamine, they take the place of joyful relationships with God and other people. They hijack the entire brain, and train it to be dependent on BEEPS for the regulation of dopamine, emotions, pleasure and pain. BEEPS attachments promise relief, but eventually leave us powerless, and make our lives unmanageable. This week's Twelve Step thought focuses on Step 1, and on helping participants understand the concepts of powerlessness and unmanageability.

Next week's lesson builds on these foundational concepts, and explains how the brain learns to flow in rhythms of joy and quiet. These are two essential skills that are developed in the first year of life – and the brain can't live without them! The lessons in weeks 3 and 4 focus on the essential task of the second year of life: learning to return to joy from negative emotions.

In addition to foundational information about the brain, this week's lesson presents two other essential elements of Thriving. The first of these elements is the joy and relationship building exercises that form a core of each Restarting lesson. For recovery to be effective, our brain must be re-trained – and that doesn't happen simply by learning new information about recovery. The exercises in Restarting are important, because they teach new joy and relationship building skills that re-train the brain. This solution-centered approach to recovery is an essential aspect of Restarting. For this reason, at least one third of each Restarting lesson is spent teaching participants simple joy and relationship building exercises that help re-train the brain. The exercises are each designed to help participants learn new right hemisphere skills that help retrain the brain – and lead to lasting recovery, sobriety and maturity.

The second element of Restarting introduced in this lesson is equally important. Learning to experience the presence of Jesus in a way that brings healing is this second essential element. Throughout this module, participants will have the

1 TRAIN YOUR BRAIN FOR A CHANGE
HOW IS THE BRAIN ORGANIZED? WHAT DOES IT NEED?

FACILITATOR NOTES

opportunity to learn and practice simple exercises that teach them to experience the presence of Jesus. These exercises are called the Immanuel Process. As participants learn to experience the presence of Jesus in painful and non-painful areas of life, they find healing that is essential for recovery from both trauma and attachments to BEEPS.

In this week's lesson, participants are introduced to the Immanuel Process in a video from Dr. Karl Lehman. In this live ministry session, a man named Rocky experiences the presence of Jesus as he works through a very painful wound in his relationship with his father. Participants will be able to watch as Rocky experiences significant healing through his interactions with Jesus. Later on, in Week 7, participants will have the opportunity to begin to learn and practice this exercise.

There are two exercises in this week's lesson. In the first exercise, participants identity a person that they appreciate and for whom they are grateful. They have the opportunity to share about an experience with this person in a small group. In the second exercise, participants will have the opportunity to answer questions about the Rocky video in small group.

Since this is the first Restarting lesson, it will be helpful to remind participants that all exercises must be done in groups of 3-5 people.

2 THE 2 SKILLS YOUR BRAIN CAN'T LIVE WITHOUT
THE RHYTHMS OF JOY AND QUIET

FACILITATOR NOTES

For a brain to be healthy, it must learn to flow in dynamic rhythms of joy and quiet. We are designed so that our brains work best when they flow smoothly and easily between these states of arousal and rest. Introducing participants to these rhythms – and how the brain learns these skills that it can't live without – is the focus of this week's lesson.

This lesson begins with a quick look at the foundational aspects of brain training that were discussed in last week's lesson. The function of the left and right hemispheres of the brain and the development of the 4 level emotional control center in the right hemisphere are reviewed. This week's lesson builds on these essential concepts, and helps us understand how we can learn to flow easily in rhythms of joy and quiet in relationships. We learn these rhythms in our first year of life.

To the brain, joy means that someone is "glad to be with me." We learn to live in joy when others who are empowered by joy are "glad to be with us." As we learned in last week's lesson, joy is communicated through non-verbal, eye-to-eye contact. This week's lesson illustrates how right hemisphere to right hemisphere joyful interactions between mother and baby help train the emotional control center of the baby's developing brain. This training in the first year of life helps develop the baby's ability to regulate dopamine and emotions for life. Photos of moms and babies building joy together help explain these concepts.

Learning to flow in rhythms of quiet is also an essential task for the first year of life. We learn to rest and quiet ourselves as mom synchronizes with our need to take a break from joyful interactions, and shares "quiet together" time with us. This interactive "quiet together" time teaches our brain to regulate serotonin effectively, and teaches us to rest. Soon, we are ready to begin another round of joy building with mom.

These cycles of alternating joy and quiet together time teach our brain to regulate dopamine (joy) and serotonin (quiet). Photos of moms and babies building joy and sharing quiet together time illustrate this process. These synchronized interactions teach our brain to regulate dopamine and serotonin – and flow easily in rhythms of joy and quiet. These rhythms give us strength and help us build bonds with others that are healthy and life giving. Our brain can't live in health without these skills.

When the brain has not learned these skills, and is unable to regulate dopamine and serotonin effectively, the effect is traumatic. Life is very painful, and the brain lacks the capacity to regulate our distress internally. As a result, the brain turns to BEEPS to help regulate emotions, pleasure and pain. BEEPS become an external means by which our brain can achieve states of pleasure or quiet. Attachments to BEEPS take the place of secure attachments and interactions with God and others.

As attachments to BEEPS grow, we literally re-wire our brains. Our brain develops neurochemical wiring that powerfully connects us to BEEPS. The longer we use BEEPS, the stronger the connections become. In the end, BEEPS leave us powerless, and life becomes unmanageable. Step 1 of the 12 Steps is again the focus of this week's 12 Step moment.

Following Ed's discussion of the rhythms of joy and quiet on this week's DVD lesson, participants have the opportunity to watch another live ministry session from Dr. Karl Lehman. In this week's session, a woman named Eileen deals with a painful memory from her past involving a wound in her relationship with her mother. As Eileen experiences the presence of Jesus in this painful area of life, she is able to make a decision to come to Him so that He can comfort her – and bring healing to her wound. It is helpful to remind participants that they will begin learning this process in Week 7 of Restarting.

This week's lesson contains 3 exercises. The first exercise helps build joy and capacity, and is similar to last week's appreciation exercise. This week, volunteers are encouraged to share about a person or experience they had in the past week for which they are grateful. The second exercise helps participants learn to quiet themselves by learning simple breathing and progressive body relaxation techniques. In the final exercise, participants will have the opportunity to answer questions about the Eileen video in a small group.

3 CALMING OUR PAINFUL EMOTIONS
RETURNING TO JOY, PART 1: SYNCHRONIZATION & NEGATIVE EMOTIONS

FACILITATOR NOTES

This is the third lesson in a four-week series that helps participants understand how the brain develops and is trained. This lesson focuses on how the brain learns to calm our painful emotions, and return us back to joy. Next week's session continues this theme, and describes Satan's two primary strategies that keep us stuck in the pain of negative emotions.

This lesson begins with a quick look back at key concepts introduced in Weeks 1 and 2. The review includes the development of the emotional control center, building joy through right hemisphere to right hemisphere communication, and the rhythms of joy and quiet. Building joy and learning to flow in rhythms of joy and quiet are essential tasks that must be completed in the first year of life.

In the second year of life, our brain is ready to learn important new skills that build on these foundations. After learning to live in rhythms of joy and quiet in our first year, the brain must now learn to return to joy from negative emotions. Learning to calm ourselves and return to joy when we experience negative emotions is our second year task, and the focus of this week's lesson.

As we learned last week, our brain only learns to flow in rhythms of joy and quiet in joyful, synchronized relationships. We learn to calm ourselves from painful emotions in the same way. To learn to return to joy from negative emotions, we need synchronized relationships with others who are empowered by joy, and glad to be with us when we are distressed. We need others to help us learn this vital skill.

In our previous lessons, we learned that joy means relationship – that someone is glad to be with us. The overwhelming intensity of negative emotions often makes it impossible for us to stay relationally connected with others when we are upset, and is one of the most painful aspects of negative emotions. When others who know how to return to joy from the negative emotions I feel, are "glad to be with me," and can stay relationally connected with me while I am upset, my brain is able to return to joy. This process of emotional synchronization trains the brain to return to joy.

By the time we are two years old, we need to have built strong connections back to joy from each of the "Big Six" negative emotions. The big six negative emotions are anger, fear, sadness, shame, disgust and hopeless despair. If our brain has not made strong connections back to joy from these negative emotions, we will get stuck in negative emotions. We won't be able to get back to joy. This means that we will not be able to stay connected relationally to others, and will be consumed with trying to make our pain stop.

Becoming stuck in negative emotions means that the brain will crave relief. Since the brain has not learned to return to joy, there is no internal pathway in the brain between negative emotions and joy. The brain remains stuck in painful emotions that it has no way to resolve internally. As a result, it will tend to use BEEPS to medicate the pain. The relationships between BEEPS and negative emotions are the focus of the 12 Step questions at the end of this chapter.

Joyful and synchronized relationships are essential to build capacity and strong connections back to joy from negative emotions. These help us learn to stay connected with others, even when we are upset. These connections help us form secure attachments with God and others who are joyful.

There are two exercises this week. In the first, participants have the opportunity to learn about synchronization through a synchronized walking exercise. In addition to being a lot of fun, it provides participants with a visible illustration of synchronization. In the second exercise, participants will explore the Big Six negative emotions as they answer the question, "Why did God give us the ability to feel negative emotions?"

4 STRATEGIES THAT KEEP YOU STUCK
RETURNING TO JOY, PART 2: CAPACITY, ATTACHMENT AND BEEPS

FACILITATOR NOTES

This is the final lesson in a four-week series that helps participants understand how the brain develops and trains in the first 2 years of life. This lesson also continues last week's discussion of how the brain learns to return to joy from negative emotions.

While last week's lesson described the synchronized brain training needed to learn to return to joy from negative emotions, this week's lesson focuses on Satan's two primary strategies that are designed to keep us stuck in the pain of negative emotions. This lesson also introduces participants to the subject of attachment styles, which will be discussed at length over the next 3 weeks. "Attachment styles" describe the type of relationships – and relationship patterns – that we typically tend to develop throughout our life. Attachment styles are the direct result of the brain training and capacity that is in place by the end of our second year of life. This lesson concludes by exploring the link between negative emotions and attachments to BEEPS.

In the first year of life, the brain is designed to build joy, and learn to flow in rhythms of joy and quiet. Joyful interactions with others who are empowered by joy teach our emotional control center to regulate dopamine effectively. This allows us to develop and live in increasing levels of joy. When others synchronize with our need to rest and share "quiet together" time with us, our emotional control center learns to regulate serotonin effectively. This teaches us to calm and quiet ourselves. As we move easily between states of joy (dopamine) and quiet (serotonin), our brain learns to internally regulate mood and emotions.

Learning to flow easily in rhythms of joy and quiet prepares our brain to tackle its important second year task, learning to return to joy from negative emotions. As we discovered last week, we learn to calm ourselves from painful emotions in synchronized relationships with others who are empowered by joy and are willing to share our distress with us while we are upset. Our brain is designed to learn to return to joy only in the context of these synchronized relationships.

There are six basic negative emotions, and learning to return to joy from each of them is our task in the second year of life. The Big Six negative emotions are: anger, fear, sadness, shame, disgust and hopeless despair. We learned last week that the brain must make strong connections back to joy from each of these negative emotions. If our brain has no pathway back to joy from any of these emotions, we will get stuck in emotional pain. When that happens, we will be unable to stay connected relationally with others, and we will be consumed with trying to make the pain stop.

As you might suspect, Satan seems to enjoy the effect that the trauma of emotional pain has on our lives. He is very interested in keeping us stuck in emotional pain – and our reactions to it. As a result, he has two primary strategies that are designed to keep us stuck in the pain of negative emotions.

The first strategy is to cause us to live our lives based on pain – and the drive to find pain relief. When we live our lives in reaction to emotional pain, our most important perceived need is eliminating, avoiding or medicating pain. We can't enjoy relationships with God or others – even when they are glad to be with us – because we are pre-occupied with finding relief for our pain.

Satan's second strategy involves causing us to live our lives from our sark (sarx.) "Sark" is a biblical term that describes the part of us that lives under the delusion that we have the capacity to decide for ourselves the right thing or wrong thing to do at any given moment. The problem with the sark is that it is always wrong! We are created to know God – not good and evil. Apart from Him, our own understanding is always insufficient to know His heart for us.

Brain training, capacity and synchronization create our ability to attach to others in relationships. Pain and sark-driven belief systems lead to a lack of synchronization, deficits in capacity – and a poorly trained brain. We live in a painful state of relational and emotional trauma.

If we have learned to flow in rhythms of joy and quiet in our first year of life, and learned to return to joy from negative emotions in our second year, we are able to develop attachments with others that are secure, joyful and life giving. Unfortunately, the opposite is also true. By the end of our second year of life, if we have not built sufficient joyful capacity,

4 STRATEGIES THAT KEEP YOU STUCK
RETURNING TO JOY, PART 2: CAPACITY, ATTACHMENT AND BEEPS

FACILITATOR NOTES

haven't learned to flow in rhythms of joy and quiet, remain unsynchronized and are unable to return to joy from negative emotions, we will develop attachments with others that are not secure, joyful or life giving. Synchronization and capacity create our attachment styles. There are four attachment styles, and these are the subject of our next three lessons.

When the brain does not have adequate pathways back to joy, it lacks the internal capacity to relieve the distress caused by negative emotions. The brain's only option is to find an external source that can reliably regulate – or medicate – emotional pain. In the quest to find an external source of emotional regulation, the brain tends to discover that BEEPS quickly and temporarily medicate pain.

Over time, attachments to BEEPS can become the primary way in which the brain learns to handle emotions that it can't regulate internally. As these attachments grow, the brain becomes wired to BEEPS as its primary source for the regulation of emotions, pleasure and pain. The wiring between BEEPS and negative emotions is part of the mental mismanagement and insanity that characterizes attachments to BEEPS. Our 12 Step moment this week focuses on Step 2.

There are two exercises in this week's lesson. In the first, participants have the opportunity to share what they learned about negative emotions from last week's lesson. In the second exercise, participants will learn to tell stories that build joy. These are called Level 4+ stories, because they involve both the control center in the right hemisphere of the brain, as well as words from the left hemisphere. This is an important and essential Restarting – and Thriving – exercise.

5 HEALTHY RELATIONSHIPS
WHAT IS SECURE ATTACHMENT?

FACILITATOR NOTES

This lesson is the first in a three-part series that is designed to help participants understand the unique development, characteristics and impact of secure, dismissive, distracted, and disorganized attachments. This week's lesson introduces participants to secure attachment, which is an essential component of all healthy relationships. This lesson also introduces participants to attachment pain, which is the type of distress we feel when our attachments are not secure.

As we learned in last week's lesson, brain training, capacity and synchronization create our ability to attach to others in relationships. If we have learned to flow in rhythms of joy and quiet in our first year of life, and learned to return to joy from negative emotions in our second year, we are able to develop attachments with others that are secure, joyful and life giving. Unfortunately, the opposite is also true. By the end of our second year of life, if we have not built sufficient joyful capacity, haven't learned to flow in rhythms of joy and quiet, remain unsynchronized and are unable to return to joy from negative emotions, we will develop attachments with others that are not secure, joyful or life giving. Brain training, capacity and synchronization lead directly to the development of consistent attachment styles.

God has created us to be able to attach securely to Him and to each other, and is totally committed to secure attachment with us. When our attachments are secure, our lives are powered by joy. We are able to synchronize with each other, bond and work together in joy, and fulfill our unique God-given purposes together. We are designed to be completely fulfilled only in joyful, secure relationships with each other.

Attachment pain is what we feel when we are not able to experience secure attachments with God and with each other. Attachment pain affects us sub-cortically at level one of our emotional control center, and is the deepest level of pain we can experience. Even though pain at this level is below our conscious awareness, it can powerfully affect every area of life.

In our previous lessons, we learned that level one of our control center helps us regulate dopamine. Appropriate regulation of dopamine is essential to feel pleasure, build joy and regulate emotional distress. Living in attachment pain means that our brain's ability to regulate pleasure and mood may be significantly impaired at its deepest and most fundamental level. As a result, the entire emotional control center is desynchronized, and this impairs our ability to regulate adrenaline and serotonin. Our brain is in a massive amount of pain. It feels like everything hurts!

When the control center is desynchronized through attachment pain, the brain is unable to regulate pleasure, pain or emotions effectively. Lacking the internal resources to resolve this incredible level of distress, the brain searches for an external source to regulate our pain. The brain may turn to BEEPS such as alcohol, drugs, food, sex, relationships, masturbation, work, gambling, rage, cutting – or any other behavior that provides some measure of relief. The greater the level of attachment pain, and the more we use BEEPS to medicate our distress, the stronger our attachments to BEEPS become. BEEPS literally hijack the attachment center at level one of our control center – and regulate our pain for us.

Because attachment pain is subcortical, it may exist for years without ever being consciously identified. Recognition and interpretation of attachment pain must be learned. One of the focuses of this week's lesson and exercises is helping participants recognize the characteristics of attachment pain – and the behaviors associated with it.

Attachment pain and attachments to BEEPS bring us to a point of absolute powerlessness in which our thinking is hopelessly toxic and our lives are completely unmanageable. None of us has the internal resources to overcome these on our own. To recover, we need a power greater than ourselves who can heal and restore our brain from the devastating effects of attachment pain and BEEPS – and who can retrain our brain as we experience and build joyful capacity with this power greater than ourselves. Jesus is the One who is best qualified and most willing to take on this task, and bring joy, healing and comfort to our lives.

This week's Twelve Step moment focuses on Step 3 in which we make "a decision to turn our will and lives over to the care of God as we understood Him." When we turn our will and life over to the care of Jesus, He attaches to us in complete and absolute joy – and our lives may never be the same again!

6 PAINFUL RELATIONSHIPS
DISMISSIVE AND DISTRACTED ATTACHMENT

FACILITATOR NOTES

tionships, and their relationship partners often feel crowded and overwhelmed. People with distracted attachment may have a series of intense – but unsatisfying relationships.

Both dismissive and distracted attachments are very painful, and continue to re-traumatize us throughout our lifespan. Persons with dismissive attachment attempt to deal with their pain by avoiding relationships. People with distracted attachment attempt to deal with pain by trying to have many intense relationships.

Unfortunately, neither one of these strategies is able to effectively address pain that exists due to a lack of brain training, joyful capacity and synchronization. These attachment styles hinder and sabotage our ability to develop secure and synchronized relationships with others that could help us develop the joyful capacity we desperately need. Our own dismissive and distracted attachment styles continue to re-traumatize us, decrease our capacity, and increase our level of pain.

As we have seen previously, when the brain is unable to regulate pain and emotional distress internally, it looks for external sources to medicate the pain. Dismissive and distracted attachments are both the cause and result of attachment pain that the brain is unable to regulate. Both of these painful attachments lead to the development of attachments to BEEPS. These attachments to BEEPS help the brain medicate emotions, pleasure and pain – and take the place of secure attachments with God and others. These attachments to BEEPS leave us more relationally isolated – which already makes the problems of attachment pain worse. This week's Twelve Step moments focus on Steps 4 and 5.

There are four exercises in this week's lesson. The first exercise reviews attachment pain from last week's lesson by asking participants to vote on their favorite attachment pain song. In the second and third exercises, participants learn to tell Level 4 non-verbal stories to illustrate dismissive and distracted attachments. You will have to stop the video to lead these exercises. In the final exercise, participants improve their ability to return to negative emotions by learning to tell a Level 4+ Return To Joy From Negative Emotions Story.

7 DISORGANIZED ATTACHMENT AND TRAUMA
TOXIC RELATIONSHIPS

FACILITATOR NOTES

This lesson is the third in a three-part series that is designed to help participants understand the unique development, characteristics and impact of secure, dismissive, distracted, and disorganized attachments. This lesson focuses on disorganized attachment – which is the most toxic of all relationship and attachment styles – and begins a two-week study of trauma. This week, participants will also have the opportunity to learn the Immanuel Process, which was first introduced in Weeks 1 and 2.

When our study began, we learned that brain training, capacity and synchronization create our ability to attach to others in relationships. Secure, dismissive, distracted and disorganized attachment styles all reflect the level of brain training we receive during our first two years of life. These attachment styles tend to be very consistent throughout our lifespan.

Secure attachments are the result of high joy capacity and synchronized bonds. Non-secure attachments are the direct result of a lack of joy capacity and synchronization – and the inability to return to joy from negative emotions. The resulting pain and distress keep us disconnected from joyful and secure attachments with God and with each other. Unless our brains are re-trained through the development of joyful and synchronized bonds with others, non-secure attachments will damage our relationships throughout our lifespan. Dismissive and distracted attachments are examples of painful attachment styles that lead to painful relationships, and both were discussed in detail last week.

This week's lesson focuses on disorganized attachment, which is the most traumatic and toxic attachment style of all. Disorganized attachment results when mom, or the primary attachment figure in an infant's life, is both a source of comfort – and a source of terror. Because the parent's behavior is frequently chaotic, disorganized and terrifying, the infant has no consistent, secure or joyful source of synchronization. It is impossible for a baby to receive comfort from – or securely attach to – mom or a primary caregiver who may at one minute appear to be loving and is the next minute physically, verbally, sexually or emotionally abusive.

As a result, the infant learns to exist in high states of arousal and fear – with no way to calm or quiet the distress. There is little joy capacity, and the control center of the brain is simply too disorganized – and untrained – to regulate emotions, pleasure or pain effectively. This resulting attachment style is called disorganized attachment.

Disorganized attachment is the most painful of all attachment styles. People with disorganized attachment have a high likelihood of having clinical problems, and are at high risk for developing attachments to BEEPS. Their relationships with peers are very difficult, and may be marked by hostility, aggression and manipulation – followed by fearful withdrawal. Lacking the ability to regulate emotions internally, persons with disorganized attachments may display intense emotional outbursts. As adults, persons with disorganized attachment may be physically, sexually, emotionally or physically abusive – or may be the victims of these kinds of abuse. Disorganized relationships are highly toxic – and excruciatingly painful.

All three non-secure attachment styles lead to the development of ongoing pain and trauma and make social relationships difficult. This makes it even more difficult to develop life-giving relationships with others who are empowered by joy. These relationships with joyful others are critical for the development of capacity, synchronized relationships and brain training, which are the things that people with non-secure attachments need the most. Because dismissive, distracted and disorganized attachment styles actually sabotage the development of healthy relationships with others, they contribute to ongoing emotional and relational trauma.

Trauma is an event or series of events that overwhelm our capacity to handle the experience. There are two types of trauma introduced in this week's lesson. "Trauma A" exists when we experience the absence of the good and necessary things that we need to develop healthy capacity. "Trauma B" exists when we experience bad things that tend to overwhelm our existing capacity. Both Trauma A and Trauma B are devastating to our lives, and will be discussed at greater length in next week's lesson.

The experience of Trauma A and/or Trauma B leaves the emotional control center in the right hemisphere of the brain in a tremendous amount of painful distress that it is unable to regulate effectively. Attachments to BEEPS that help the brain

7 DISORGANIZED ATTACHMENT AND TRAUMA
TOXIC RELATIONSHIPS

FACILITATOR NOTES

artificially regulate emotions, pleasure and pain tend to be the tragic result. This week's 12 Step moment emphasizes the relational nature of the Twelve Steps, and the need for balance in our recovery from both trauma and BEEPS.

Following Ed's discussion of disorganized attachment and trauma in this week's lesson, participants have the opportunity to watch another live ministry session from Dr. Karl Lehman. In this week's session, a woman named Crystal encounters the presence of Jesus as He helps her heal from significant trauma and attachment pain concerning her father. Following the video, participants will have the opportunity to begin learning to experience the presence of Jesus as they learn the Immanuel Process.

There are 3 exercises in this week's lesson. The first lesson is an appreciation exercise. In the second, participants will learn to tell Level 4 stories about distracted attachment. In the final exercise, participants have the opportunity to start learning the Immanuel Process, which is designed to help them begin to experience the presence of Jesus.

8 TRAUMA, HOPE AND RECOVERY
TRAUMA

FACILITATOR NOTES

The focus of this week's lesson is on helping participants understand the devastating impact of trauma on the brain. This lesson also expands last week's Immanuel Process exercise to help participants learn to experience the presence of Jesus in areas of life that have not felt peaceful. Experiencing the presence of Jesus in painful areas of life brings hope – and recovery – to those of us whose lives have been devastated by trauma.

As we have seen in our study, the level of brain training, capacity and synchronization that we develop in the first two years of life create our ability to attach to others in relationships. These first two years are essential for the development of joyful capacity and synchronized bonds that help the control center in the right hemisphere of the brain regulate emotions, pleasure and pain effectively. When we have developed strong joy capacity and synchronized bonds in the first two years of life, our emotional control center is healthy, and is well able to regulate our emotions, pleasure and pain. This allows us to form secure attachments with others that are life giving, and further enhance our level of brain training through the development of joyful and synchronized bonds.

On the other hand, the lack of joyful and synchronized bonds in our first two years of life leaves our control center unable to regulate emotions, pleasure and pain effectively. The lack of joyful capacity, synchronization and brain training leaves us stuck in pain – and leads to the development of non-secure attachments with others. Our painful dismissive, distracted and disorganized attachments make it very difficult for us to form life-giving relationships with others that could help retrain our brains through the development of joyful and synchronized bonds. Moreover, since these non-secure attachments tend to damage relationships throughout our lifespan, they actually make our attachment pain worse. We live in a state of chronic and ongoing trauma and lack the secure attachments that could help us heal and retrain our brain.

Trauma is an experience or series of experiences that overwhelm our capacity. In last week's lesson, we found that "Trauma A" exists when we experience the absence of the good and necessary things that we need to develop healthy capacity. We are easily overwhelmed when we have experienced Trauma A, because we don't have the capacity to handle the normal pain and distress of life. "Trauma B" exists when we experience bad things that tend to overwhelm our existing capacity. With Trauma B, we experience a level of pain that our control center is not able to regulate. The combination of Trauma A and Trauma B together is devastating to our lives, relationships and brain.

Trauma A and Trauma B can lead to severe disruption of communication between the left and right hemispheres of the brain, and desynchronize communication between different levels of the control center in the right hemisphere. When we suffer such a massive shutdown of communication in the brain, the right amygdala at level two of the control center assumes control of the brain until the distress has passed. This means that we enter a state of fear-based thinking, and tend to function according to very primitive fight/flight impulses. We may also enter a very destructive state called dissociation, in which all possible circuits in the brain are shut down in an attempt to conserve energy and survive the trauma.

The experience of Trauma A or Trauma B leaves our brain unable to regulate positive or negative emotions, pleasure and pain effectively. When the brain is unable to regulate its distress internally, it searches an external source of attachment to help it regulate our pain. As we have seen, attachments to BEEPS temporarily medicate pain for the brain. In the end however, attachments to BEEPS create increasingly destructive levels of pain, and further desynchronize the control center. This week's 12 Step moment emphasizes the relational nature of the 12 Steps and recovery – and highlights our need for balance in recovery from both trauma and BEEPS.

There are two exercises this week, and both are based on the Immanuel Process exercise from last week's lesson. In the first exercise, participants have the opportunity to share about a moment in the past week in which they experienced the presence of Jesus. The second exercise allows participants another opportunity to learn and practice the Immanuel Process. This time, participants will learn to move with Jesus into previously non-peaceful places of life, and have the opportunity to experience his presence with them in a way that brings healing, joy and peace.

Please be aware that any discussion of trauma can be painful for participants. For this reason, you will need to be very sensitive and encouraging as you facilitate this group.

9 LEAVING CODEPENDENCY BEHIND
BEEPS MEDICATE TO REGULATE PART 1: SECURE ATTACHMENTS, IDENTITY & INTERDEPENDENCE

FACILITATOR NOTES

This week's lesson begins a two part series that helps participants understand how the development and growth of attachments can lead to either healthy interdependent relationships or harmful attachments to BEEPS. This week's lesson focuses on the growth of life-giving interdependent relationships that help us leave codependency behind! Next week's lesson will describe the growth of attachments to BEEPS that re-wire the brain and lead to harmful dependency.

This lesson begins with a discussion of BEEPS, and helps participants recognize that healthy interdependence and harmful dependence both begin with attachments. Healthy attachments lead to the development of strong, joyful capacity and the ability to return to joy from negative emotions. From these, a strong, joyful individual identity develops, and this allows for the later formation of a strong, healthy group identity. A strong, healthy individual and group identity is essential for the development of healthy interdependence.

As we have learned in previous lessons, the level of brain training we experience in our first two years of life leads to the development of either secure or non-secure attachments. Strong joyful capacity, the ability to quiet ourselves effectively, and the ability to return to joy from negative emotions lead to the development of a secure attachment style. Our control center in the right hemisphere of the brain is able to regulate emotions, pleasure and pain effectively. Secure attachments are the foundation for healthy relationships.

The development of an effective control center and secure attachments allow us to develop an identity that is strong, healthy and joyful. As we grow, the development of a healthy individual identity allows us to form a joyful and strong group identity. The combinations of a healthy control center, secure attachments, and strong individual and group identities allow us to form relationships with God and others that are characterized by healthy interdependence.

The growth of attachments that lead to healthy interdependence follow a predictable course of growth through three distinct stages. The progressive stages that describe the development and nature of attachments are intensity, intimacy and exclusivity. This chapter describes the characteristics of attachments that lead to the development of healthy interdependent relationships at each of these stages of growth. As we will see in next week's lesson, the development of harmful dependency from attachments to BEEPS can also be described through the stages of intensity, intimacy and exclusivity. This week's Twelve Step moment focuses on Steps 6 and 7.

Following Ed's discussion of identity, attachment and healthy interdependence, participants will see another video from Dr. Karl Lehman. In this video, a woman named Maggie describes an exciting Immanuel Process moment with Jesus.

There are three exercises in this week's lesson. The first exercise follows up with last week's Immanuel Process, and asks volunteers to share about a moment they had this week in which they experienced the presence of Jesus. In the second exercise, participants learn to tell Level 4+ and Level 4 stories about healthy interdependence. The final exercise for the week is a short discussion of Maggie's Immanuel Process moment. There is also an optional exercise included with this week's lesson. It uses a song to help participants explore the relationship between two people when BEEPS are involved in their attachment.

10 ATTACHMENTS THAT KILL: HOW ADDICTIONS RE-WIRE YOUR BRAIN
BEEPS ATTACHMENT & IDENTITY MEDICATE TO REGULATE PART 2: HARMFUL DEPENDENCY

FACILITATOR NOTES

This week's lesson concludes a two part series that helps participants understand how the development of attachments can lead to either healthy interdependent relationships or harmful attachments to BEEPS. Last week's lesson focused on the growth of life-giving interdependent relationships that help us leave codependency behind. This week's lesson describes the growth of attachments to BEEPS that re-wire our brain and lead to harmful dependency, attachment pain and death.

We learned last week that both healthy interdependence and harmful dependence begin with attachments. The foundation of healthy interdependence begins in the first 2 years of life. In these early years, strong joyful capacity, the ability to quiet ourselves effectively, and the ability to return to joy from negative emotions help train the control center of our brain to regulate emotions, pleasure and pain effectively. This effective brain training leads to the development of an attachment style that is secure. Our secure attachment style allows us to build an individual and group identity that are strong. A strong identity leads to developing life-giving relationships that with healthy interdependence.

The foundations of attachments to BEEPS that lead to harmful dependency also have roots in the first two years of life. The lack of joyful capacity and synchronized bonds in these early years of life leaves our control center unable to regulate emotions, pleasure and pain effectively. Our lack of capacity, synchronization and brain training leaves us stuck in pain and leads to the development of non-secure attachments with others. Dismissive, distracted and disorganized attachment styles are traumatic and lead to the development of an individual and group identity that is rooted in pain.

Throughout this process, the brain lacks the training, capacity and synchronized bonds to resolve our increasing level of attachment pain. The brain simply does not have the internal resources to do the job. Our non-secure attachments keep us from forming secure attachments and joyful bonds with others that could help re-train our brain. Our attachment pain remains unchecked and unregulated.

As a result, the attachment center of the brain searches for a source of reliable attachment to help regulate this devastating internal distress. Since some BEEPS stimulate feelings of arousal and pleasure and others tend to quiet and calm us, BEEPS offer the control center of the brain an artificial and external source of regulation for distressing emotions, pleasure and pain. Moreover, since BEEPS stimulate the dopamine sensitive pleasure center of the brain, they mimic the effects of secure and joyful relationships. In this way, attachments to BEEPS hijack the attachment center of the brain and lead to harmful dependency.

Attachments to BEEPS follow a predictable course of growth through three distinct stages and lead to harmful dependency. The progressive stages that describe the development and characteristics of attachments to BEEPS are intensity, intimacy and exclusivity. This week, we will discover how harmful dependency develops as our attachments to BEEPS grow through each of these three stages. We will also find out how BEEPS alter our control center so that our brain becomes more responsive to BEEPS and less responsive to other joyful attachments that could re-train our brain to build joy and capacity. BEEPS are truly a jealous lover!

As we have seen, attachments to BEEPS tend to develop from inadequate relational brain training, non-secure attachments, trauma and a painful individual and group identity. We live with high levels of attachment pain, emotional distress and the experience of ongoing trauma. To make matters worse, attachments to BEEPS significantly damage our relationships with God and others, and this only increases our levels of attachment pain and distress.

For recovery to be effective, it must be relational. The brain only learns to build joyful capacity, quiet itself and regulate emotions, pleasure and pain in the context of secure attachments with God and others who are empowered by joy. As a result, a joyful healing community – a spiritual family – is an essential aspect of recovery. Such a community offers us the best hope for being able to identify and address our attachment pain, trauma, painful identity and attachments to BEEPS.

As we are able to build new relationships with others who are glad to be with us, our brain can learn new skills and be re-trained in joy! We can build the capacity to examine issues related to trauma and non-secure attachments, and build

10 ATTACHMENTS THAT KILL: HOW ADDICTIONS RE-WIRE YOUR BRAIN
BEEPS ATTACHMENT & IDENTITY MEDICATE TO REGULATE PART 2: HARMFUL DEPENDENCY

FACILITATOR NOTES

long-term sobriety. We can begin to experience the healing presence of Jesus and allow Him to heal our attachment pain and trauma. Our attachments and identity can be rooted in life-giving joy, and not the pain of our past. Sobriety and the development of long-term maturity are possible. Our relationships will become a place of healing and growth – not a place of pain and separation.

In this week's Twelve Step moment, our focus is on Steps 8 and 9. These steps can help us begin to restore relationships that have been damaged as a result of our attachments to BEEPS if we can learn to work them as part of a healing community.

There are three exercises in this week's lesson.

The first is an appreciation exercise about an experience with healthy interdependence. This exercise helps build joy and capacity. Joy capacity is needed before beginning our discussion of attachments to BEEPS. In the second exercise, participants will tell a Level 4 story that describes what attachments to BEEPS look like. The final exercise combines a relaxation exercise with an Immanuel Process moment.

11 RECOVERING OUR LOST IDENTITY
MATURITY AND CAPACITY PART 1: WHAT IS MATURITY?

FACILITATOR NOTES

This week's lesson begins a two-part discussion of maturity and capacity that will conclude in Session 12. These two lessons bring together concepts from all previous Restarting lessons to describe the process of ongoing recovery and maturity. As we mature, we recover from painful life trauma and attachments to BEEPS. The development of ongoing maturity suggests a recovery that is Thriving!

The goal of this week's session is to help participants answer the question, "What is maturity?" By helping participants answer this vital question, the lesson will empower them to begin to recover their original identity that was lost due to the pain of trauma and BEEPS. Next week's lesson defines the stages of maturity, and helps participants understand what the tasks and needs are at each stage.

Maturity and growth are a lifetime process. As we mature, we discover that we are increasingly becoming the people that God created us to be. We maximize our identity, increase our God-given potential and expand our capacity to the fullest extent possible. We are becoming the people that we always wanted to be.

The development of ongoing maturity is not a gift. It does not grow on trees or happen by accident. Maturity – and recovering our identity – happens because we become intentional about growing our own maturity. This process involves life-giving relationships with family and community that are empowered by joy.

As we engage with community, we are able to receive – and give – appropriately. As we have seen in previous lessons, joyful capacity and synchronized bonds help build secure attachments. These attachments are foundational for the recovery of our personal & individual identity, healthy interdependence and the development of ongoing maturity.

In the absence of joyful capacity, synchronization and secure attachments, many of us were unable to discover and live from our true identity. As our individual and group identity became increasingly centered in pain, our true self became increasingly lost to us. BEEPS became the only way we were able to cope with our pain and "hold it together" enough to function. By helping us temporarily cope with our pain and "hold it together" BEEPS produced the appearance of stability and maturity. Unfortunately, this pseudo-maturity did not produce genuine growth and maturity in us. Instead, it created a "house of cards" that failed under stress and kept us stuck in cycles of chronic immaturity.

This week's Twelve Step moment describes Steps 10, 11 and 12, which are called "maintenance steps." Practicing these steps as part of a mature and life giving community can help us grow in sobriety and maturity.

There are two exercises in this week's lesson. In the first exercise, participants have the opportunity to answer the question, "What do I want my new life in recovery to look like?" In the second exercise, participants will have the opportunity to learn a scripture meditation exercise to help them experience the presence of Jesus.

12 THE BLUEPRINT FOR A NEW YOU!
MATURITY AND CAPACITY PART 2: THE STAGES OF MATURITY

FACILITATOR NOTES

This week's lesson concludes a two-part discussion of maturity and capacity that began last week. Last week's lesson introduced the concept and characteristics of maturity, and helped participants answer the question, "What is Maturity?" This week's session helps participants develop a clear picture of the resources and tasks they need to grow through each stage of maturity. It helps them understand "the big picture of life," develop a working blueprint for growth and assess their current level of maturity. Finally, the lesson helps participants understand the next step of growth they can take through the Thriving: Recover Your Life program.

This lesson begins by identifying the six stages of maturity, which are unborn, infant, child, adult, parent and elder. The development of maturity as we grow through these stages is a lifetime journey in which we are gradually becoming more fully alive. We discover that we are increasingly living from our heart as the unique person that God designed – and as the person we have always wanted to be.

Recognizing the needs and tasks we have at each stage of maturity helps us develop this "big picture of life." Defining the specific needs and tasks at each level of maturity is a primary focus of this lesson. By understanding our needs in each stage, we can become intentional about finding the people, community and resources that are essential to our journey. By understanding our tasks associated with each stage, we can learn to accept the responsibilities – and challenges – that empower our growth. Finally, by recognizing the limitations inherent in each stage of maturity, we can avoid taking on responsibilities that exceed our level of maturity. This helps keep us safe as we grow.

This lesson also discusses the pitfalls of ignoring maturity. The failure to mature keeps us stuck in cycles of pain, trauma, immaturity and BEEPS. It also leads to repeated personal and relationship failure – and makes life generally frustrating. We remain unsatisfied, overwhelmed – and immature. To help participants who are beginning to identify areas of immaturity, trauma and BEEPS in their own lives, this lesson asks the question, "What do I need to restore missing maturity – and what is the next step in my recovery?" This lesson helps participants proactively answer this question in two ways. First, it presents an overview of the entire Thriving: Recover Your Life program, and introduces them to the next Thriving module. Second, this lesson allows students the opportunity to evaluate their level of maturity by taking a maturity assessment test.

Belonging is the second module in the Thriving: Recover Your Life program. One simple way in which participants can develop maturity and continue their recovery from trauma and BEEPS is by becoming part of Belonging. Belonging is designed to build on the foundation that participants received in Restarting, and to help them maintain continuity in their recovery. In Belonging, participants have the opportunity to become part of a joyful recovery community and learn to practice some of the 19 brain skills that they need to Thrive.

The final exercise in this week's lesson consists of a maturity assessment. In this assessment, participants have the opportunity to complete an evaluation that focuses on the tasks essential for the development of an infant or child level of maturity. This assessment helps participants recognize their existing level of maturity. By recognizing gaps in maturity, participants can identify the needs, tasks and the resources they need to grow and develop ongoing maturity. Belonging, and the entire Thriving: Recover Your Life program are designed to serve as resources to help build maturity, joyful community – ongoing recovery from the pain of trauma and BEEPS.

This week's Twelve Step moment focuses on the importance of working the Steps in a joyful, healing and mature community. This helps keep our recovery in relational balance, and leads to the development of ongoing maturity.

There are two exercises this week. The first is an appreciation exercise in which volunteers can share about a person in their life who models healthy maturity. In the second exercise, participants have the opportunity to complete their maturity assessment. It is important for participants to recognize that this assessment is for their use only. It does not have to be shared in small group or with anyone else.